BEST PRACTICE
FINANCIAL
MANAGEMENT

Six Key Concepts for Healthcare Leaders

Third Edition

BEST PRACTICE
FINANCIAL
MANAGEMENT

Six Key Concepts for Healthcare Leaders

Third Edition

Kenneth Kaufman

ACHE Management Series

Health Administration Press

Chicago, Illinois

Your board, staff, or clients may also benefit from this book's insight. For more information on quantity discounts, contact the Health Administration Press marketing manager at 312/424-9470.

Library of Congress Cataloging-in-Publication Data

Kaufman, Kenneth V.
     Best practice financial management: six key concepts for healthcare leaders/
        Kenneth Kaufman.
        p. cm.
     Rev. ed. of: Finance in brief. 2nd ed. 2003.
     Includes bibliographical references and index.
     ISBN-13: 978-1-56793-259-1
     ISBN-10: 1-56793-259-2
     1. Health facilities—Business management. 2. Health facilities—Finance.
3. Health services administrators. I. Kaufman, Kenneth V. Finance in brief. II. Title.

RA971.3 .K383 2006
362.1068—dc22   2006041181

The paper used in this publication meets the minimum requirements of American National Standards for Information Sciences—Permanence of Paper for Printed Library Materials, ANSI z39.48–1984.

Health Administration Press   Acquisitions manager: Audrey Kaufman
A division of the Foundation of   Project manager: Amanda Bove
     the American College of   Layout editor: Robert Rush
     Healthcare Executives
One North Franklin Street, Suite 1700
Chicago, IL 60606-3424
(312) 424-2800

Contents

Preface

FOR MANY YEARS now I have written articles and books on the general topic of healthcare finance. It turns out that finance is like medicine; everyone knows they need it to stay well (or get well), but nobody really enjoys taking it. More than six years ago Kaufman, Hall & Associates, Inc., the American College of Healthcare Executives, and Health Administration Press joined forces to help the healthcare industry "take its finance medicine." The result of this effort was the first edition of *Finance in Brief: Six Key Concepts for Healthcare Leaders*, published in 2000. The content of *Finance in Brief* was strong medicine, but the easy-to-understand, question-and-answer format made the book highly readable (as finance books go) and the message much easier to swallow.

The second edition, published in 2003, was considerably enhanced by new material on estimating risk and budgeting and three case studies that illustrated financial planning, capital allocation, and strategic budgeting in practice. I wish to extend thanks to key leaders at each of the three healthcare organizations that assisted in the presentation of the case examples. We have respected the confidentiality of each organization to ensure the candor, accuracy, and illustrative value of each business case.

This third edition benefits from a number of significant changes, including a revised title that more accurately indicates the publication's scope—*Best Practice Financial Management: Six Key Concepts for Healthcare Leaders*—a new accessible format, revised and additional material to enhance each chapter, and a completely new chapter, "Achieving the Right Capital Structure." A special thanks to Jason H. Sussman, partner of Kaufman, Hall & Associates, Inc., for his contribution of chapters 4 and 5.

The staff of Health Administration Press, especially Audrey Kaufman, have once again proven to be a pleasure to work with. Being an author is not easy, but Health Administration Press makes the writing process as easy as it can be.

Once again, Nancy Gorham Haiman has served as consultant and editor to the project. Nancy is a consummate professional, and the third edition greatly benefited from her desire that, first and foremost, *Best Practice Financial Management* should communicate effectively to the widest readership possible.

Kaufman, Hall & Associates, Inc. is a firm that values new ideas and the practical application of those ideas. Needless to say, many of those ideas have found their way into the third edition. In this regard, the book's content, and its clear point of view, should certainly be seen as a collective effort of all the staff and professionals of the firm.

And last, but never least, thanks to my wife Barbara. Nothing I have accomplished, this book or otherwise, could have been done without her.

Introduction

Publication Goals

Best Practice Financial Management: Six Key Concepts for Healthcare Leaders provides healthcare executives and board members with concise information on what is often considered a daunting subject: best practice healthcare financial management using a corporate finance–based approach.

Intended to help the wary "over the hump," the book introduces six key principles critical to the effective financial management of healthcare organizations: the capital management cycle, creditworthiness, integrated strategic and financial planning, capital allocation, strategic budgeting, and capital structure management. With a basic understanding of these principles, healthcare executives and trustees will be equipped with a common language and approach to high-quality financial decision making.

The need for this book is more pressing than ever. Healthcare has become a highly competitive business. A healthcare organization's strategic mission must be supported by financially sound practices and a business plan that generates a positive bottom line. Once the sole province of *Fortune 500* companies, the language of corporate finance must now be understood by all individuals at the decision-making table in healthcare organizations nationwide.

This book is geared to executives, senior managers, and trustees of all types of healthcare organizations, including hospitals (not-for-profit and for-profit); health systems; and long-term care, behavioral health, ambulatory care, home care, and other healthcare facilities. It is written in a user-friendly way. Formal financial training is not required; a receptive mind is required.

This third edition represents a significant revision from the first and second editions published in 2000 and 2003, respectively, under the title *Finance in Brief: Six Key Concepts for Healthcare Leaders.*

With a revised title to more accurately indicate the publication's scope—*Best Practice Financial Management: Six Key Concepts for Healthcare Leaders*—the third edition reflects new developments in the field and an enhanced level of understanding of what it takes to captain healthcare organizations through financially challenging waters. New information and up-to-date statistical data have been added to all chapters. One completely new chapter, Concept Six: "Achieving the Right Capital Structure," addresses the critical importance of effective capital structure management to increased capital access, added flexibility, and lower overall cost of capital. This chapter replaces a previous chapter on risk and simulation analysis, the key material of which has been incorporated in other chapters, as appropriate.

Examples or case studies describe the experiences of actual healthcare organizations in implementing best practice credit analysis and financial planning, capital allocation, and budgeting. These appear at the end of Concept Three, Concept Four, and Concept Five, respectively. We hope leaders of all types of healthcare organizations use the lessons learned to jump-start the implementation of best practice approaches.

Contents Overview

Organized in an easily accessible format, each of the six chapters covers a basic principle of corporate finance.

Concept One, "Managing the Capital Cycle," describes why healthcare executives and board members need to worry about corporate finance and introduces the capital management cycle. It outlines the four control points of healthcare financial management and why organizations frequently fail to achieve their strategic financial goals. It also describes the six essential characteristics of financially successful organizations.

Concept Two, "Analyzing and Boosting Creditworthiness," addresses why creditworthiness is important to healthcare organizations. It outlines factors influencing access to capital in the current healthcare environment and the key organizational determinants of creditworthiness, as defined by the capital markets. This new information derives from recent in-depth interviews with analysts in the agencies that rate healthcare credits, insurers that offer healthcare bond insurance, and investors in healthcare debt issues. The chapter also provides the key ratios that should be used to analyze creditworthiness and describes how to perform a financial credit analysis. Key strategies for credit fitness and key information reviewed by the agencies during the rating process are outlined.

Concept Three, "Integrated Strategic and Financial Planning," describes the leadership required for effectively integrated planning, the integrated planning process, and the components of a high-quality plan. It presents the organizing principle that should be used throughout the process and takes readers through key process steps. Steps include identifying and selecting strategic initiatives based on solid market data and consideration of risk, estimating capital requirements through a multiyear financial plan that links strategies to capital requirements, determining capital sources, and determining the level of profitability required to close the capital shortfall. It also describes the techniques leaders can use to test the reasonableness of their goals and projections and enhance the effective implementation of the integrated plan. A case example at the end of the chapter describes one organization's implementation of the best practice planning process.

Concept Four, "Allocating Capital," describes the characteristics of a best practice capital allocation process. It addresses who should be responsible for the process, the key steps involved, and strategies to ensure its successful implementation. It also describes specific goals of project analysis and provides basic information on quantitative techniques that can be used to analyze a potential investment, including net present value analysis. The chapter also describes methods for ranking and selecting projects. A detailed example at the end of the chapter illustrates how one organization implemented a corporate finance–based capital allocation process.

Concept Five, "Strategic Budgeting," covers a best practice budgeting process that directly connects the organization's mission and objectives to the day-to-day efforts of its staff. It describes the eight key steps of budgeting that start when leaders define the organization's strategic and financial goals and interactively gain buy-in for identified operating targets from operating staff. It outlines how these targets then drive the development of the initial or first-pass budget, which is reviewed by department managers and finalized by finance staff. The chapter also provides information on the time frame for the budgeting process and the attributes of tools critical to its success. A case example at the end of the chapter describes how one organization implemented a best practice strategic budgeting process.

Concept Six, "Achieving the Right Capital Structure," describes the benefits of a strategic and proactive approach to capital structure management. It includes information on the major categories of traditional and off-balance-sheet nontraditional debt vehicles available to healthcare organizations and the criteria organizations should use to select the most appropriate vehicle. The chapter also provides guidance on achieving the right mix of fixed-rate and variable-rate debt and describes the risks and benefits of interest-rate swaps and other derivatives that can be used within an overall debt portfolio to maintain maximum financial flexibility, lowest possible interest costs, and acceptable levels of risk.

The "Concluding Comments" section summarizes the need for a corporate finance–based approach to healthcare financial management and provides a synopsis of the key managerial issues covered in this book.

A bibliography guides readers to relevant literature. Although the list of publications is by no means complete, it serves as a starting point for additional information.

A subject index provides readers with easy access to information covered in the book.

CONCEPT ONE

Managing the Capital Cycle

THERE ONCE WAS a lord of a castle. He lived in the Land of Three Rivers. His castle was a nice, comfortable one, and the surrounding lands produced food aplenty for the lord and his people. In spite of prosperity, however, the lord hungered for additional lands. He annexed many fiefdoms within a very short time—some peaceably, some not. Most of the fiefdoms were poor and needed the lord's help for food and know-how about developing their lands. "No problem," thought the lord. "Within a year or two, the fiefdoms will be able to feed and fend for themselves and return goods to the Land of Three Rivers." Meanwhile, the lord developed the home castle and sent knights to conquer new lands.

As the lord expanded his empire, several of the new fiefdoms started to run out of food. They simply could not make their land productive as quickly as the lord expected. Unable to feed their own people, they certainly could not return food to the lord's castle to help feed others. Other fiefdoms followed suit. Within a year, the lord's empire had crumbled. He sold off the fiefdoms in faraway lands. Unable to feed his own people, the lord put his castle up for sale and moved away from the Land of Three Rivers in disgrace.

To healthcare executives who have been in the industry for a decade or more, the story will sound familiar. This medieval allegory recounts Allegheny Health Education and Research Foundation's (AHERF) plight in 1998. Although occurring nearly ten years ago, the story is still relevant—

I

particularly in view of the many noncore business ventures, such as health plans, physician practices, and capitation, hospitals pursued as fiefdoms in the late 1990s. The plight of AHERF illustrates the consequences associated with not understanding the "circle game" involved with the capital cycle. This game balances business strategies with financial ability. When played properly, it results in solid financial performance; when played poorly, it results in inadequate financial performance or worse. Because its plan was built on the assumption that each of the acquired hospitals or entities could be made profitable within a short time, AHERF stumbled. When a number of the hospitals performed poorly for multiple years, requiring a continued infusion of cash for operations, the structure built by AHERF's lord crumbled. A similar thing happened to other healthcare organizations when physician practices or health maintenance organizations (HMOs) didn't perform as expected. Why?

Going round and round in the circle game requires effective leaders who are comfortable "playing the game," "talking the talk," and "walking the walk." Understanding the application of corporate finance principles is key. So is the proper management of the capital cycle. Quite simply, these were absent in the Land of Three Rivers.

Importance of the Principles of Corporate Finance

Leaders of healthcare organizations need to know more than a little about finance to effectively manage their organizations. Chief executive officers (CEOs) of *Fortune 500* companies like General Electric (GE) and Microsoft certainly rely on corporate finance principles to manage the strategic and financial risk of their organizations. Why should things be different in the healthcare field?

In fact, because of constrained reimbursement and increasing competition, costs, regulation, and complexity, healthcare leaders must be well versed in finance. No longer can they afford to treat finance as a stepchild. Minor decisions do not exist in the financial arena. All decisions have major implications for an organization's success and even, perhaps, survival. Once the domain of the finance department, an understanding of corporate finance principles is now the responsibility of the organization's entire management team.

Healthcare boards of trustees must also understand these principles. The Sarbanes-Oxley Act of 2002, which technically applies only to the corporate world at this time, has increased the sense of urgency about boards having financial expertise in the not-for-profit world as well. The act requires the boards of public companies to meet stringent self-auditing and other governance requirements. Many healthcare boards are voluntarily using key Sarbanes-Oxley guidelines to ensure their compliance with fiduciary responsibilities.

Being a trustee today simply demands a higher level of financial knowledge and a common language in boardrooms, as trustees and management teams make decisions with major and long-term strategic and financial implications. Not surprisingly, the most recent survey of the not-for-profit industry indicates that board education and board performance are highly correlated. Boards that invest significant dollars in education receive higher overall performance ratings, including strategic direction-setting and financial oversight (The Governance Institute 2005).

In healthcare more has changed in recent years than just reimbursement levels. In fact, economic incentives have undergone a revolution. As the intensity of change increases, the time between significant changes appears to be decreasing. Gone are the years of pursuing strategic missions centered on improving health in local communities without financially sound business plans that generate profitable bottom lines. The hospital industry has crossed over from a public, mission-driven operating model to an operating model that closely resembles that of corporate America. Board members and senior executives must now demonstrate the ability to balance organizational values and fulfillment of mission with solid financial practices that ensure continued competitive financial performance.

The Capital Management Cycle

The capital management cycle or strategic capital cycle, a core concept of corporate finance, is the circular path involved in managing the flow of capital from the development of market- and mission-based strategic plans that require funding through financial implementation of selected strategic options and back to the planning process. The capital cycle includes three essential components that are both reinforcing and interrelated:

1. a continuous, integrated, *strategic financial planning* process that effectively balances an organization's strategies with its financial capabilities;
2. a *capital structure* process that is appropriate to the organization's current financial and credit position; and
3. a *capital allocation* process that permits the organization to prioritize capital spending decisions in a manner that will improve the services provided while protecting long-term financial capacity.

Figure 1-1 illustrates the cycle. Managing the capital cycle starts and ends with the strategic financial planning process; this stage of the cycle is covered in Concept Three. Capital allocation is covered in Concept Five. Concept Six addresses the management of capital structure.

Managing the capital cycle is absolutely essential to the positive financial performance of healthcare organizations. Senior leaders must understand how to achieve best practice cycle management and must understand the technical and mathematical relationships between cycle components. Success or failure with one component affects success or failure in other parts of the cycle.

For example, without thorough financial planning, an organization will not know whether it is making the best use of available resources funded and allocated through the capital structure and capital allocation processes. Similarly, without access to required debt and equity capital, ensured through effective capital structure management, an organization's strategic competitive plan is "dead on arrival."

Faced with competitive pressures, organizations may be tempted to leapfrog over cycle steps, moving directly from strategic planning to implementing strategic options, for example. However, the long-term financial success of complex healthcare delivery organizations depends on developing and maintaining a financial plan, and carefully and deliberately allocating capital.

To succeed in a competitive environment, the capital cycle must be competently managed. This ensures that the organization is positioned to deliver capital resources when and where they are needed to achieve strategic objectives. It also enables an organization to expand and renew capital capacity. Clearly, the long-term success of any organization depends on its ability to

FIGURE 1-1. The Capital Management Cycle

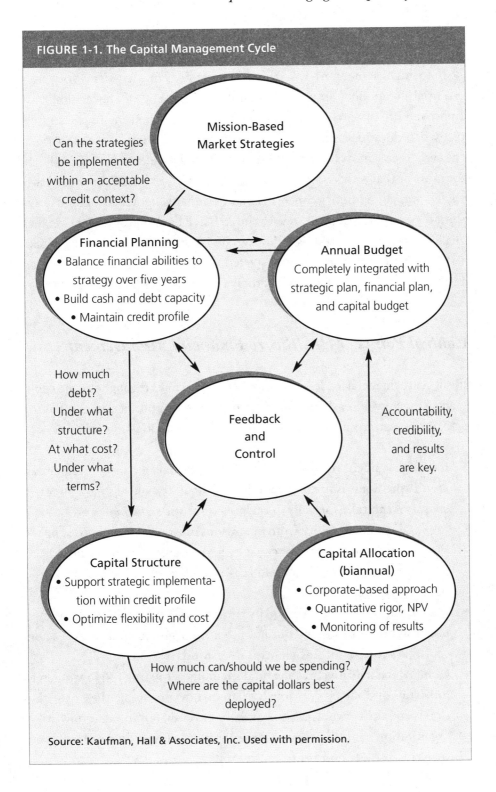

Source: Kaufman, Hall & Associates, Inc. Used with permission.

make capital investment decisions that will eventually add to and enhance its future capital capacity.

The management of a healthcare organization's *credit position* is an essential component in the successful management of the capital cycle. Improved creditworthiness provides positive momentum to all strategic plans; deteriorating credit has the opposite effect. Throughout the 1980s and the early 1990s, most hospitals were accustomed to relatively easy credit and, for most of that period, low-cost debt. As a result, organizational creditworthiness was not a priority concern. Credit standards tightened significantly in the late 1990s, at least partly due to the AHERF bankruptcy and the financial challenges faced by hospitals following the Balanced Budget Act (see Sidebar 1-1). Credit has only very recently started to ease for many healthcare organizations. For more information on creditworthiness, see Concept Two.

Control Points of Healthcare Financial Management

Healthcare financial leaders coordinate four variables throughout the capital management cycle: cash, profitability, debt, and capital spending. A description of these points of control and their relative relationships follows:

- *Cash*: How much "free cash" should be on the balance sheet? Remember, creditworthiness is highly dependent on liquidity, and cash is a direct source of capital, especially in the not-for-profit environment.
- *Profitability*: Profitability from operations must be sufficient to support the required amount of debt capacity and ensure appropriate liquidity. The appropriate level of debt and cash will determine long-term profitability requirements.
- *Debt*: Debt should be governed by the following philosophy: Not too much, as everyone knows, but not too little. Unfortunately, this is a concept that is often not sufficiently understood.
- *Capital spending*: How much capital spending is too much? How much is too little? The answers obviously relate to how profitable the organization is and the appropriate mix of debt and cash. A reminder: how an organization allocates its capital spending dollars can be more important than the absolute number of dollars spent.

SIDEBAR 1-1. The Continuing Impact of Allegheny Health Education and Research Foundation's (AHERF) Bankruptcy

The impact of AHERF's $1.4 billion bankruptcy filing in 1998 continues to be felt in the healthcare industry. Repercussions include the following:

- Access to capital tightened dramatically (and only now is showing some signs of improvement).

- Terms for capital have also tightened. Restrictive covenants—particularly those related to liquidity—have become standard. Greater debt security, often in the form of mortgages and revenue pledges, is now required.

- Access to bond insurance fell dramatically in the late 1990s and early 2000s and only now, with the reentry of two major bond insurers into the healthcare bond-insurance marketplace, is showing signs of improvement. The dollar volume of insured debt inched past the dollar volume of uninsured debt in 2004, but there were more than twice as many uninsured than insured debt issues (Thomson Financial and Citigroup 2004). This indicates that uninsured issues were much smaller on average.

- Creditors are demanding greater scrutiny of hospital finances. The capital marketplace is requiring tax-exempt healthcare organizations to report just like corporate borrowers through the nonprofit version of a 10-K and 10-Q (Wareham 2001). Quarterly financial reporting has become standard for new healthcare bond issues. Voluntary disclosure has increased. Since the collapse of Enron and the passage of the Sarbanes-Oxley Act of 2002, there is also increased regulatory focus on independence of the corporate audit, compliance with ethical codes, use of gifts and retirement funds, and accuracy of financial statements and disclosures.

- Increased liquidity in the form of cash has become the "insurance policy" demanded of healthcare organizations by the capital market. The "days cash on hand" ratio, *the* critical measure of liquidity, has steadily increased during the last decade.

Based on its current financial position and external operating environment, each healthcare organization has an optimal solution set for these variables. This solution set is the preferred quantitative outcome between and among the points of control. Solving for the solution set through algebraic calculations is not required of senior management. Rather, the management team must ensure that such quantification is accomplished, that the results and interrelationships between variables are well understood by the team and board members, and that the financial performance of the organization is safely managed within identified constraints. Figure 1-2 illustrates the points of control of healthcare financial management.

Characteristics of Financially Troubled Organizations

Organizations that are financially troubled fail to prosper because one or more of three basic "financial pathologies" are present in their boardrooms:

1. All forest—no trees
2. All trees—no forest
3. Management of incremental financial events

In the *all forest–no trees* pathology, the board wants the big picture but doesn't want to be bothered with the day-to-day details of financial management. "Details are what management does," says the all forest–no trees board. A global understanding of what the organization is trying to accomplish is not accompanied by respect for the planning and implementation of actions that will make the goals happen. Also lacking is an assurance that the critical financial responsibilities of the organization are being handled properly on a daily basis.

For example, the board understands the big-picture results of declining investment earnings because of stock market losses. However, having not come to grips with its full responsibility in the trees arena, it doesn't consider whether the organization's financial managers have taken steps to ensure that the pension fund is properly capitalized. In fact, this issue is never discussed. The frame of the puzzle is assembled, but the pieces cannot possibly fit into a whole.

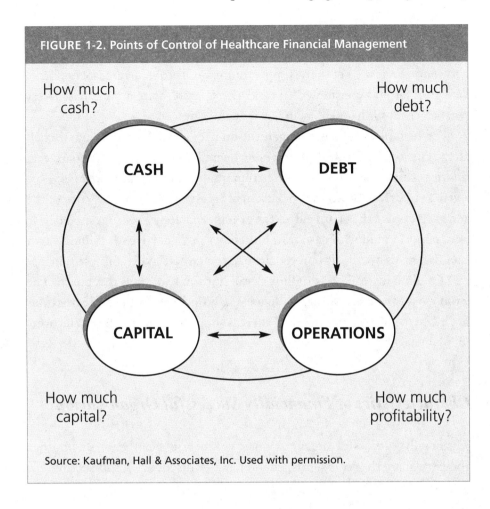

FIGURE 1-2. Points of Control of Healthcare Financial Management

How much cash?

How much debt?

CASH

DEBT

CAPITAL

OPERATIONS

How much capital?

How much profitability?

Source: Kaufman, Hall & Associates, Inc. Used with permission.

In the *all trees–no forest* pathology, which is perhaps the most prevalent of the three pathologies, the board lacks a clear understanding of the organization's overall strategic financial goals and objectives and concentrates only on the details of day-to-day management. During board meetings, simple agenda items degenerate into 45-minute conversations on such subjects as "how to reduce receivables." Board members appear to be itching to come to work and actually run the organization. Without an aerial strategic financial vision, the puzzle pieces have no frame. Board members and management cannot possibly interact in an intelligent and systematic way to establish and meet financial objectives.

A large portion of U.S. healthcare organizations exhibit the third pathology—*management of incremental financial events*. Like the second pathology, it is characterized by the absence of a comprehensive strategic financial road map that describes what the organization is trying to accomplish and how it will get there. Opportunities and problems are isolated from one another and considered to be truly separate, unrelated issues. Every financial event is handled in an incremental way.

For example, perhaps an organization needs to achieve ten major goals in the course of a fiscal year to meet its overall financial target. A board that addresses financial events in an incremental fashion cannot articulate the overall objective. As progress or lack of progress toward reaching each of the ten goals occurs, the board judges the events separately. Project A should have generated $2 million of cash flow but comes in at just over $1 million. "Not bad," says this board, "It's pretty close to the target." Next, project B brings in $3 million instead of $5 million. "Still not too bad," says this board. The problem is this: If each program sequentially underperforms, and no actions are taken to balance the equation, there is simply no way to achieve the overall financial target.

Characteristics of Financially Successful Organizations

Financially successful organizations, whether in healthcare or another industry, share the six essential characteristics discussed in this section.

Sound and financially literate leaders

Financially successful organizations have leaders who can envision, engage, and execute. Senior leaders have the capacity to envision the organization's future. They know how to move a group of people forward on a common mission and deliver results that exceed rather than meet expectations. They respond quickly and appropriately to a rapidly changing environment and at the same time address new realities in internal operations.

Financially successful organizations most often have CEOs who are financially literate, financially interested, and financially responsible. They recognize the need for and importance of financial leadership. They set concrete goals and objectives and lead the team toward goal attainment. Such organizations also generally have a chief financial officer (CFO) who is a strategic leader and an essential member of the executive team. The CFO is often viewed both internally and externally as the number two executive in the organization.

The boards of financially successful organizations govern around explicit expectations and metrics and are guided by an attitude that senior management will deliver expected results on a consistent basis. The board's comprehensive view of the organization's overall financial target enables it to manage all events toward reaching that objective. The whole is clear; so are the pieces that make up the whole. If one area underperforms, the board knows that other areas must do better than forecasted or new revenue-generating programs, cost controls, or exit strategies must be added to the puzzle. Real accountability exists between the board and senior management.

Commitment to corporate finance principles and a single financial perspective

In successful organizations, corporate finance principles are an integral component of management's philosophy. The organization, the board, and the management team buy into and faithfully maintain a single financial perspective. This holistic approach organizes decision making by the entire leadership group around one and only one financial philosophy. The principle that has proven most effective is as follows:

Financial performance must be sufficient to meet the cash flow requirements of the strategic plan and, at the same time, maintain or improve the financial integrity of the organization within an appropriate credit and risk context.

Board members and executives use this principle to guide their decision making and measure their success. Their goal is to ensure that the organization's financial condition at the end of each fiscal year is at least as good as and hopefully better than it was at the beginning of the year. Every financial decision is made with this principle in mind.

For example, if someone suggests making an acquisition costing $30 million, every member of the board and management team asks the question, "Will this acquisition allow us to better meet the cash flow requirements of our strategic plan and secure the competitive position of the organization?" If the answer is no, the leaders engage well-entrenched second thoughts about whether the acquisition is appropriate.

The organizing principle is written down to ensure common understanding. It is given to every board member, senior executive, and middle manager, and its implications are discussed in full during orientations for new board members or executives.

Commitment to financial learning

Leaders of financially successful organizations understand that financial leadership is possible only through acquiring the necessary financial knowledge. In many organizations, a strong continuing education process is necessary to teach and reinforce critical corporate finance skills. Sound financial management becomes a reality when a basic finance skill set is learned by managers deep into and throughout the organization.

A planning philosophy and process

A planning philosophy and planning processes provide the platform for both long-term strategic and day-to-day operating decisions. The planning philosophy frames the business vision, strategy, financial goals and objectives, and tactics to achieve results. The financial plan is an integral part of management's control of complex decision making and its direction of operating results. All major strategic opportunities are vetted through the financial plan. The capital allocation planning process is formal, serious, highly defined, and disciplined. The process identifies projects worthy of funding and funds those projects. Technical analysis is first class and performed throughout the organization.

Disciplined execution of plans

Senior management commands operations with a liberal dose of the right attitude. Day-to-day work in financially successful organizations is performed well. Managers follow best practice in revenue cycle and expense-control management. Compromises that damage financial performance are avoided.

Active management of capital structure and respect for capital markets

Through the active management of capital structure, financially successful organizations are continuously seeking ideas and approaches to lower the total present value costs of existing and future debt service. These organizations view their credit ratings as an asset and as a mechanism to improve access to capital and lower overall capital costs. They give high priority and attention to managing their relationships with the rating agencies, bond insurers, and other capital market constituents.

How much finance do healthcare leaders need to know? More than they needed to know 15 years ago, or 10 years ago, or even 5 years ago. Clearly, to go round and round successfully in the healthcare circle game, they need to know more finance than ever before.

References

The Governance Institute. 2005. *Raising the Bar: Increased Accountability, Transparency, and Board Performance*. San Diego, CA: The Governance Institute.

Thomson Financial and Citigroup. 2004. Data provided to author.

Wareham, T. L. 2001. "Strategies for Navigating the Healthcare Credit Market." *Healthcare Financial Management* 55 (4): 55.

CONCEPT TWO

Analyzing and Boosting Creditworthiness

UTTER THE WORDS "credit rating," and most people shudder. Images spring to mind of credit card statements outlining obscene interest rates for unpaid bills or, worse yet, of an embarrassing moment when credit was denied while trying to buy the latest software at the local computer store. Indeed, as an indication of America's preoccupation with credit ratings, various Internet service providers let customers access their credit rating from home pages to learn what the agencies are reporting about the status of their personal credit. Our sense of worth seems to be tied to our line of credit.

Why Creditworthiness Matters

Is this angst different for a healthcare organization? Not really. An organization's long-term competitive position today is substantially dependent on its ability to raise affordable capital in the debt markets. An organization's board and management team must attain and maintain a minimum credit rating that permits the organization to effectively compete in its marketplace. Simply stated, credit ratings matter. Why?

First, creditworthy organizations have improved capital market opportunities. One such opportunity is *access to credit enhancement* such as bond

SIDEBAR 2-1. What Is a Bond Rating?

A bond rating is a credit agency's assessment of the ability and willingness of an issuer of debt to make full and timely payments of principal and interest on the debt security over the course of its maturity. Bond ratings are surveyed at regular intervals throughout the life of the bonds to reflect internal and external factors that may affect the credit profile and to assure investors of the accuracy of the rating at any given time.

Each rating agency uses a slightly different rating system, as shown below (from high rating to low rating for investment-grade bonds):

Fitch Ratings	AA, AA-, A+, A, A-, BBB+, BBB, BBB-
Moody's Investors Service	Aaa, Aa1, Aa2, Aa3, A1, A2, A3, Baa1, Baa2, Baa3
Standard & Poor's	AA+, AA, AA-, A+, A, A-, BBB+, BBB, BBB-

Each agency offers noninvestment grade ratings as well. Ratings are issuer specific, meaning that they are assigned by credit agencies based on an evaluation of factors affecting the debt issuer.

Sources: Moody's Investors Service. 2005a. *Not-for-Profit Healthcare: 2005 Outlook and Medians.* New York; Standard & Poor's. 2005a. *U.S. Not-For-Profit Healthcare 2005 Median Ratios.* New York; Fitch Ratings. 2005a. *Healthcare Rating Actions for the Nine Months Ended Sept. 30, 2005.* New York.

insurance or a letter or line of credit. By purchasing bond insurance or a line of credit, an organization in the "A" rated or better category essentially can "buy up" to a higher credit rating. A higher rating means lower interest costs. A small decrease in the interest rate multiplied out over the life of the bond can mean significant savings. A single-notch drop in a bond rating by Fitch Ratings, Moody's, or Standard & Poor's (S&P) (see Sidebar 2-1) can mean a significant difference in the price of capital.

Second, creditworthy organizations also have *access to both taxable and tax-exempt debt*. Taxable debt may be required for certain programs or services that don't qualify for tax-exempt debt. Organizations with a strong credit rating ("A" rating or better) may want to exercise the option of taxable debt for investments such as medical office buildings or joint-venture ambulatory facilities. Creditworthy organizations can also access derivative options such as interest rate swaps, caps, and other means or mechanisms to reduce over-all interest rate costs and risk exposure.

Third, creditworthy organizations enjoy *less restrictive bond document covenants*, which give them the full benefit of financial flexibility. Lower-rated organizations are held to different standards that limit their flexibility to pro-tect investors.

Fourth, creditworthy organizations also experience *lower costs associated with issuing their bonds*. Many of the large investor groups, funds, and insur-ance corporations that normally buy tax-exempt hospital bonds are precluded from buying debt beneath the "A"-rated category. Hence, the pool of potential investors for "BBB" bonds, for example, is much smaller than that for higher-rated bonds. Selling to a larger pool simply takes less time and energy and results in lower issuance costs. Because of the lower risk associ-ated with issuing bonds for a creditworthy organization, insurance premiums are lower, as are letters and lines of credit from banks as well as underwrit-ing and remarketing charges. In addition, organizations with impeccable credit can often issue their debt without setting aside a *debt-service reserve fund*. Organizations with deteriorating credit will often be required to estab-lish such a fund by setting aside at least a year's worth of principle and inter-est payments in an escrow account that cannot be accessed. This increases the amount of the borrowing, thereby increasing total principle and inter-est payments over the life of the bond.

Fifth and finally, creditworthy organizations are *market consolidators*. Organizations with the highest credit ratings are the most attractive part-ners to those with lower ratings. Such organizations offer excess capital capacity and lower capital costs. In the current healthcare environment, strong organizations are consolidating markets by acquiring or merging with weaker competitors that are often no longer able to compete because of a lack of access to cost-effective capital. As one expert notes, "Winners in the competition for capital are hospitals and systems that can invest in their future. Capital-poor provider organizations will be forced to sit on the side-lines in a growth era, unable to expand or upgrade facilities" (Coile 2002).

SIDEBAR 2-2. Why Credit Ratings Matter

Creditworthy organizations—organizations with high credit ratings—have improved capital market opportunities, including
- access to credit enhancement;
- access to taxable or tax-exempt debt;
- access to derivative options; and
- less restrictive bond document covenants.

Creditworthy organizations have a lower cost of capital because they experience
- lower interest rates (the interest rate differential between higher and lower credits can be [and have been] very significant depending on market conditions); and
- lower issuance costs related to insurance premiums, letters/lines of credit, and underwriting/remarketing.

Creditworthy organizations are market consolidators:
- Nationwide, organizations with the highest credit rating have been the most attractive partners, have excess capital capacity, and exhibit the lowest cost of capital.

Source: Kaufman, Hall & Associates, Inc. Used with permission.

A summary of why credit ratings matter appears in Sidebar 2-2.

External Factors Influencing Ratings and Access to Capital

Numerous pressures currently influencing the healthcare industry affect the credit ratings of healthcare providers and thus their access to capital. Many of these pressures are systemic and include the following:

- Impact of federal and state fiscal issues on Medicare and Medicaid programs, resulting in possible future reduction of provider payments
- Rising bad debt and charity care associated with providing care to an increasing number of uninsured and underinsured patients
- Slowing of the growth in commercial health insurance payments resulting from cost shifting related to consumer-directed health plans

- New financial and operational challenges associated with aging facilities and information technology (IT) infrastructure
- Increased salary, wages, and benefits expenses resulting from tighter labor markets
- Increasing costs associated with regulatory compliance and losses from physician practice acquisitions and other noncore acquisition strategies
- Increased competition due to industry consolidation, and introduction of for-profit operators and physician-sponsored niche ventures in the most profitable service areas

The *financial effects of government efforts to reduce healthcare spending* will undoubtedly become more severe during the next decade. The evaporation of the short-lived federal budget surplus of 1998 to 2001 has been followed by a period of rapidly mounting deficits. According to Congressional Budget Office (2006) projections, this situation will be reversed from a $318 billion deficit in 2005 to a $73 billion surplus in 2015. In an effort to make this happen, Medicare and Medicaid spending, which makes up more than one-quarter of the federal budget, will come under heavy Congressional scrutiny and will likely be reduced wherever possible. Per-capita state Medicaid spending for healthcare is likely to decline as well. Such reductions will have a significant impact on not-for-profit hospitals, as Medicare and Medicaid typically account for about 50 percent of total revenue.

The economic downturn in 2001 and continued hefty insurance premium increases since that time are forcing many small employers to withdraw healthcare benefits from the list of employee offerings. Significantly more Americans are going without health insurance or are underinsured. This has increased the proportion of uncompensated care provided by hospitals and bad debt expense because consumers default on bill payment at a rate higher than commercial insurers (Moody's Investors Service 2005a).

Revenue increases from commercial insurers are likely to slow during the next decade as consumer-directed health plans become increasingly popular among employers. These plans shift "first dollar" costs to consumers in the form of high deductibles and copayments. Utilization, particularly in the outpatient arena, could decline as consumers delay or forego discretionary diagnostic and treatment services.

After the Balanced Budget Act of 1997 and up through 2001, many hospitals and health systems reduced *capital spending* to respond to often declining operating cash flow. During this period, capital spending increased only 1 percent per year. This spending restraint has led to pent-up demand for capital to replace or renovate aging facilities; purchase new IT, digital radiology, and physician order-entry systems; and meet various emergency readiness requirements. Accordingly, hospital and health system CFOs indicated that their organizations expected to increase capital spending from 2002 through 2007 on an average of 14 percent annually (Healthcare Financial Management Association 2004, 11). Actual total aggregate dollar spending for capital has indeed increased since 2002 (Moody's Investors Service 2004), and major facility expansion and other expenditures continue to be planned and implemented.

Continued *staffing shortages* are making it hard for some hospitals to meet the increasing demand for inpatient beds and emergency services. The aging baby boomer population is fueling rising demand at a time when most hospitals are experiencing capacity constraints. Staffing shortages are likely to continue during the next 20 years and will not be limited to nursing, but will include therapists, pharmacists, laboratory and radiological technologists, and billing/coders. Many hospitals are paying higher wages to attract and retain staff or are using temporary agency nurses to fill vacancies, at a cost of twice that of staff nurses. In addition to shortages, hospitals are likely to be faced with workers who require new skills and training to provide rapidly changing technology–based diagnostic and therapeutic services (O'Neil 2005).

Providers will need to dig deeper into their pockets to cover the costs associated with *regulatory compliance*. Increased government and regulatory focus on quality measures and patient safety will spur the need for major IT investment by healthcare organizations. Specific IT needs focus on electronic medical records and an improved clinical management system that aids decision making, thereby enhancing patient safety and care quality. Because of its ability to position organizations for the future, credit rating agencies are paying particularly close attention to hospital investment in IT. Notes one agency:

> As we move into 2006 and beyond, the ability to improve quality and its measurement is expected to be an increasingly important business driver. Providers that successfully transition to a culture of evidence-based medicine and outcomes measurement, and that can demonstrate high quality, can be expected to demand and receive the best pricing from managed care companies, and

to use this information in appealing directly to consumers for this business (Standard & Poor's 2005b).

Integration strategies of the late 1990s became disintegration strategies in the new millennium, as providers rethought their organizational structures to ensure the financial health of core businesses. Nonperforming non-acute assets, such as physician practices, home health, and insurance plans, have mostly been restructured or divested.

Increasing competition from physicians and for-profit companies is of concern to hospitals and health systems nationwide and to the agencies that rate their debt issues. These competitors are developing outpatient and freestanding specialty facilities, such as ambulatory surgery centers and specialty hospitals. Not-for-profit hospitals are reacting by pursuing their own facilities or joint ventures to stem the flow of dollars from profitable service lines, such as orthopedics and cardiology.

Organizational Determinants of Creditworthiness

During the past decade, rating agencies have shifted their focus from a micro-analysis of organizations as stand-alone entities to a broader macroanalysis of organizations as part of complex regional and national healthcare systems. The emphasis in individual credit analyses is on how an organization has positioned itself in the past and is positioning itself for the future. Notes one agency:

> [W]ithout the inclusion of a fiscally sound business plan that generates a profitable bottom line, the ability [of healthcare providers] to pursue their founding mission will be limited. Consequently, we have shifted our analysis to focus on providers' strategic initiatives and business plans for the future—what they need to do to adjust to upcoming changes—namely, how to survive with less cash flow in a continually changing environment (Moody's Investors Service 2000).

Sidebar 2-3 outlines information reviewed in the rating process.

The rating agencies and their capital market colleagues, including institutional investors and bond insurers, conduct sophisticated and in-depth

SIDEBAR 2-3. Information Reviewed in the Rating Process

- *Organization, governance, and management*: Brief history, description of services, corporate legal structure, parent/subsidiary relationships and governance, board structure and members, and management biographies

- *Strategic/business position*: Patient origin, market share, demographics, income levels, competition, payers (mix, relations, and contracts), employers, unemployment rates, charity care, business/program/service mix, inpatient and outpatient utilization statistics (for the past five years and year-to-date interim figures with the prior year's comparable period), competitive costs/charges

- *Financial status*: Annual audited financial statements for the past five years and year-to-date interim statements with the prior year's comparable period; financial feasibility study, or management projections, especially for new money issues; sources and uses of funds statement; five-year financial projections with assumptions and cash flow statement; consolidated debt-service tables and schedule (including bonded debt, guaranties, and capital leases); schedule of principal and interest payments for both proposed and outstanding debt, including capital leases and non indenture debt; and pension expense

- *Medical and nursing staff*: Number, specialties, age, percentage of admissions, recruitment and retention plans and tools, nursing staff turnover and vacancy rates, salary and benefits structure for nursing staff, board certification of physicians, and union negotiation information, as applicable

- *Relevant business documents*: Preliminary official statement/prospectus, including Appendix A, strategic plan, capital plan, financial plan, budget for coming year, investment/debt policies, and swap documents

- *Relevant legal documents*: Master trust indenture, trust indenture, loan agreements, accreditation report, and offering documents

Sources: Fitch Ratings. 2005b. *Rating Process for Nonprofit Healthcare Credits*. New York; Moody's Investors Service. 2000. *An Updated Approach to Rating Not-for-Profit Healthcare Organizations*. New York; Standard & Poor's. *Not-for-Profit Healthcare: Inside the Rating Process*. New York.

research and analysis. They thoroughly assess relevant data to evaluate whether the organization understands its marketplace challenges and opportunities and is able to identify financially viable and competitive strategies to be successful. The results of their analyses can be material to bond rating, insurance, and lending decisions (Grube and Wareham 2005).

The agencies look at what they call "strategy" as being critical to current rating assessments of not-for-profit healthcare entities. Strategy encompasses key creditworthiness factors broadly categorized as governance and management, market and strategic position, and financial performance and debt position. Each is described below.

Governance and management

An organization's *governance and management functions* are highly scrutinized to establish and ensure accurate credit ratings. Effective leadership is critical to strong financial performance, which, in turn, is critical to creditworthiness. "[A] strong management team enables an organization to reach its full potential within the limitations or opportunities of fundamental market characteristics," notes one rating agency (Moody's Investors Service 2005b).

Good managers and board members can make things happen; ineffective managers and board members cannot. Finding the right people is particularly critical for providers during periods of rapid change. Rating agencies are interested in determining whether management has developed or hired people with the new skills and understanding to cope with new marketplace challenges and whether the organization has modified its operations to meet the challenges. Given the age of many top executives, succession planning is important.

Board members are often assessed to determine their ability to balance market and growth opportunities with sensible financial performance. They must be capable of high-level strategic thinking, but equally importantly, they must be able to link strategy to financial projections and analysis. Notes one rating agency analyst, "Board and management ability to integrate strategy and finance will influence a rating" (Goldstein 2005). A healthy respect for the capital markets and recognition of the importance of preserving credit quality are essential. Sidebar 2-4 outlines key characteristics of successful management teams.

> **SIDEBAR 2-4. Characteristics of Successful Hospital Management Teams**
>
> - Mix of newer and tenured members to provide broad and diversified experience levels
> - Cohesive approach to managing operations with all senior members being able to articulate key financial and strategic objectives
> - Balance of mission and financial strength with recognition of the need to satisfy various constituent groups while allocating limited resources and generating adequate cash flow
> - Identification of potential operating risks and challenges and articulation of strategies to address the issues
> - Timely implementation of strategies, including reversals of strategies if warranted
> - Establishment of conservative and consistent accounting practices and financial policies
> - Development of a long-term strategic and financial plan with realistic assumptions and the flexibility to respond to unforeseen events
>
> Source: Moody's Investors Service. 2005b. *Indicators of Successful Management for Not-for-Profit Hospitals*. New York. Used with permission.

Market and strategic position

Market and strategic position involves assessing the organization's market strength and competitive differentiation, both of which are critical to long-term competitive financial performance. Is there significant competition? As competition increases, so does the risk to the organization's financial position. Is the organization able to compete for clinical services, physicians, and care settings in a market with expanded geographic coverage?

Other key questions include the following: How attractive is the organization to payers? How able is it to provide a full spectrum of services in the lowest possible cost setting (i.e., generally in outpatient sites)? Is the organization able to compete as a cost-effective provider? How effectively does the organization compete for physician loyalty to obtain patient referrals? What strategies and methods does the healthcare organization use to link the medical staff and their patients to the hospital and to increase the organization's primary care base? Is the local economy growing? How do the state's policies, legislation, and regulations affect the provision of care?

Data required to answer all of these questions are not "nice-to-know" information but rather "need-to-know" information for the capital markets.

Financial performance and debt position

A healthcare organization' creditworthiness is determined by its *financial performance*. Financial performance and particularly *debt position* indicate an organization's ability to repay debt. Critical mass and consistency are important in the current healthcare environment. Credit agencies analyze systemwide rather than entity-specific operations through review of consolidated financial information. The focus is on cash flow generated from core operations and on the key ratios that incorporate cash flow. These factors go to the heart of the assessment of credit risk.

Multiyear financial planning and financial projections that are linked to the concrete initiatives described in the organization's strategic plan are strongly preferred by the rating agencies and bond insurers. For many capital players, the absence of such financial projections that prove affordability completely discredits an organization's strategy (Grube and Wareham 2005). How cash balances are invested is important, as are the organization's dependence on nonoperating income to bolster profit margins and ability to duplicate or exceed the current year's financial performance.

Dozens of factors are relevant to financial performance; the challenge is to select those most indicative of the organization's financial strengths and weaknesses. The following ten indicators are key measures used in many effective financial analyses:

Profitability Indicators
1. *Operating margin* reflects the profitability of an organization from its active patient care and related operations.
2. *Excess margin* reflects profitability from operations and includes revenue and expense from nonoperating activities, such as investment earnings and philanthropy.
3. *Operating earnings before interest, depreciation, and amortization (EBIDA)*

margin provides a good look at an organization's ability to generate enough cash to meet interest and principal payments on debt.

Liquidity Indicators

4. *Days cash on hand,* probably the most important credit ratio in use today, reflects the number of days of cash set aside by the organization to support operating expenses if revenue stream were to be reduced or eliminated.
5. *Cash-to-debt ratio* measures the availability of an organization's liquidity to pay off existing debt.
6. *Cushion ratio* compares the organization's free cash to its annual debt service—higher numbers are better than lower ones.

Debt Indicators

7. *Debt-service coverage ratio* measures the ability of an organization's cash flow to meet its debt-service requirements.
8. *Debt-to-capitalization ratio* indicates how highly leveraged, or debt financed, the organization is—the higher the capitalization ratio, the higher the risk.

Other

9. *Average age of plant* provides a relative measure of the age of the physical facilities and provides insight into the organization's future capital needs.
10. *Capital spending ratio,* a relatively new metric, assesses capital spending as a percentage of EBIDA or total revenue.

Each indicator can be expressed as a ratio (see Table 2-1).

Sample financial factors tracked by each rating agency appear as Tables 2-2, 2-3, and 2-4.

Key Reasons for Credit Rating Upgrades and Downgrades

Rating agencies revise a credit rating, either upward or downward, when an event or combination of events have weakened or strengthened an organization's ability to repay its debt obligation. In some cases, unexpected occurrences or developments, such as an earthquake or flood, have

TABLE 2-1. Key Creditworthiness Ratios

Indicator	*Financial Ratio*
Operating margin	$$\dfrac{\text{Total operating revenue} - \text{Operating expenses}}{\text{Total operating revenue}}$$
Excess margin	$$\dfrac{\text{Income from operations} + \text{Nonoperating revenue}}{\text{Total operating} + \text{Nonoperating revenue}}$$
Operating EBIDA margin	$$\dfrac{\text{Operating income} + \text{Interest} + \text{Depreciation} + \text{Amortization}}{\text{Total operating revenue}}$$
Days cash on hand	$$\dfrac{\text{Cash} + \text{Marketable securities} + \text{Board-designated funds} \times 365}{\text{Total operating expenses} - \text{Depreciation} - \text{Amortization}}$$
Cash-to-debt ratio	$$\dfrac{\text{Cash} + \text{Marketable securities} + \text{Board-designated funds}}{\text{Long-term debt} + \text{Short-term debt}}$$
Cushion ratio	$$\dfrac{\text{Cash} + \text{Marketable securities} + \text{Board-designated funds}}{\text{Maximum annual debt service}}$$
Debt-service coverage ratio	$$\dfrac{\text{Excess revenue over expenses} + \text{Depreciation} + \text{Interest} + \text{Amortization}}{\text{Annual debt service}}$$
Debt-to-capitalization ratio	$$\dfrac{\text{Long-term debt (less current portion)}}{\text{Long-term debt (less current portion)} + \text{Unrestricted net assets}}$$
Average age of plant	$$\dfrac{\text{Accumulated depreciation}}{\text{Annual depreciation}}$$
Capital spending ratio	$$\dfrac{\text{Capital expenditures (additions to property, plant, and equipment)}}{\text{Depreciation expense}}$$

Source: Kaufman, Hall & Associates, Inc. Used with permission.

TABLE 2-2. Moody's Investors Service: Freestanding Hospital & Single-State Healthcare Systems

Healthcare Medians by Rating Category, 2004 [1]

	All Ratings	Aa	A	Baa	Below Baa
Sample	387	49	180	130	28
Financial Performance ($000)					
Net patient revenues	282,321	772,599	312,337	169,927	138,744
Total operating revenue	331,918	846,262	339,657	185,975	143,068
Interest expense	4,934	11,588	5,296	3,576	3,176
Depreciation and amortization expense	16,855	45,282	18,777	10,193	6,477
Total operating expenses	300,991	808,827	336,259	188,528	137,953
Income from operations	5,453	32,612	7,600	2,143	(701)
Excess of revenue over expenses	13,862	65,980	17,338	5,811	(1)
Net revenue available for debt service	36,341	121,510	40,834	19,216	8,745
Operating cash flow	26,744	83,972	32,077	15,851	7,816
Debt service	8,565	18,064	9,452	6,673	5,549
Additions to property, plant and equipment	24,262	86,553	28,535	11,970	5,750
Balance Sheet ($000)					
Unrestricted cash and investments	114,244	521,496	147,380	55,197	21,485
Restricted cash and investments	1,899	11,196	1,882	1,038	816
Net fixed assets	151,622	451,866	177,985	96,673	57,396
Long-term debt	122,574	351,731	131,628	80,089	50,547
Short-term debt	0	0	0	0	0
Total debt	124,333	351,731	131,628	80,089	52,297
Debt service reserve and Debt service funds	5,407	3,350	4,506	7,037	5,790
Net debt	111,046	339,069	120,899	71,945	49,525
Unrestricted fund balance	168,503	710,420	215,517	89,870	21,778
Key Ratios					
Operating margin	2.0%	4.1%	2.6%	1.1%	(0.6%)
Excess margin	4.5%	7.7%	5.2%	3.1%	0.1%
Operating cash flow margin	9.0%	11.2%	9.5%	8.1%	5.9%
Return on assets	4.1%	5.8%	4.7%	3.0%	0.1%
Annual debt service coverage (x)	4.1	8.0	4.7	3.2	1.7
Maximum annual debt service coverage (x)	3.8	5.6	4.1	3.2	1.9
Current ratio (x)	1.9	1.8	2.0	2.0	1.6
Cash on hand (days)	146.3	235.0	166.0	108.0	50.6

Continued

Cushion ratio (x)	12.6	23.1	15.0	8.8	3.3
Cash-to-debt	98.3%	160.1%	118.6%	70.8%	39.6%
Accounts receivable (days)	51.4	53.5	51.4	51.3	50.3
Average payment period (days)	57.9	63.2	55.5	59.1	66.8
Debt-to-capitalization	40.8%	32.0%	37.7%	48.7%	73.5%
Debt-to-cash flow (x)	3.9	2.8	3.7	5.2	7.4
Bad debt as a percent of net patient revenue	6.1%	5.9%	5.8%	6.5%	7.1%
Average age of plant (years)	9.7	9.0	9.6	9.9	14.5
Capital spending ratio (x)	1.3	1.5	1.4	1.2	0.7

[1] Financial data is based on a sample size of 387 hospitals, excluding multi-state hospital systems. Ratings as of 6/30/05.

Source: Moody's Investors Service. 2005. *Not-for-Profit Healthcare: 2005 Outlook and Medians*. New York: Moody's Investors Service, August. Used with permission.

been material enough to warrant a rating change. Moody's Investors Service (2002) published a list of common reasons behind recent rating changes, excerpts of which follow.

Top 5 reasons for a rating upgrade

1. *Improving financial performance*: The successful combination of revenue growth and expense management, as evidenced by improving financial performance and debt indicators

2. *Market share gains*: The ability to translate market gains or clinical reputation into demonstrative financial gains, such as improved payer contracts

3. *Significant economic event, such as the discontinuation of problematic business ventures*: Closure or restructuring of money-losing ventures and cash proceeds on the divestiture improve cash flow and leverage indicators

4. *Growth in unrestricted liquidity*: Cash growth and the maintenance of higher cash levels through successful receivables management and profitable operations, which enhance liquidity and are stabilizing factors

5. *Favorable market characteristics*: Factors such as location in an economically vibrant service area and the absence of material competition

Top 5 reasons for a rating downgrade

1. *Material escalation in debt burden*: Signifies an elevated risk profile unless the organization has been able to demonstrate a near-term proportional increase in cash flow

TABLE 2-3. Standard & Poor's: Not-for-Profit Heathcare Medians, 2004
Median Ratios of Stand-Alone Hospitals: 'AA' and 'A' Categories

	AA	AA-	A+	A	A-
Sample size	14	18	47	70	69
Average daily census	381	285	234	183	144
Statement of Operations					
Net patient revenues (mil $)	563.9	359.5	304.5	221.3	154.9
Salaries and benefits/net patient revenues (%)	56.4	51.7	51.3	50.2	53.0
Bad-debt expense/total operating revenues (%)	3.3	5.1	5.8	5.1	6.1
Maximum debt service coverage (x)	5.5	4.4	4.2	4.0	3.5
Maximum debt service/total operating revenues (%)	2.9	3.2	3.2	3.1	3.4
EBIDA (mil $)	82.2	60.2	40.2	31.1	19.5
Non-operating revenues (%)	4.4	2.3	2.3	1.8	1.7
EBIDA margin (%)	15.5	13.9	12.8	12.8	11.5
Operating cash flow margin (%)	10.7	11.9	9.9	11.1	9.7
Operating margin (%)	3.8	4.8	3.4	3.2	2.9
Profit margin (%)	8.6	7.0	6.0	4.9	4.4
Capital expenses/depreciation and amortization expenses (%)	181.3	174.1	171.8	140.9	137.6
Balance Sheet					
Average age of net fixed assets (years)	8.7	8.5	9.6	9.1	9.6
Cushion ratio (x)	34.1	23.1	15.4	13.8	12.0
Days cash on hand	383.0	228.0	193.0	195.0	153.0
Days in accounts receivable	55.1	51.1	52.4	54.2	53.1
Cash flow/total liabilities (%)	22.9	21.0	19.7	17.8	18.0
Unrestricted cash/long-term debt (%)	216.7	156.8	131.9	118.2	111.2
Long-term debt/capitalization (%)	26.1	30.3	34.2	35.2	34.9
Payment period (days)	74.0	61.5	63.0	53.0	55.8

Median Ratios of Stand-Alone Hospitals: 'BBB'

	BBB+	BBB	BBB-
Sample size	71	59	55
Average daily census	117	112	71
Statement of Operations			
Net patient revenues (mil $)	116.3	111.0	64.8
Salaries and benefits/net patient revenues (%)	52.4	53.2	53.6
Bad-debt expense/total operating revenues (%)	5.2	4.9	5.8

Continued

Maximum debt service coverage (x)	3.0	2.8	2.4
Maximum debt service/total operating revenues (%)	3.8	3.6	4.2
EBIDA (mil $)	14.1	12.3	6.6
Non-operating revenues (%)	1.4	1.3	0.9
EBIDA margin (%)	11.4	10.1	9.2
Operating cash flow margin (%)	10.1	8.7	8.1
Operating margin (%)	2.6	1.4	1.0
Profit margin (%)	4.4	2.7	2.3
Capital expenses/depreciation and amortization expenses (%)	136.6	124.1	102.9
Balance Sheet			
Average age of net fixed assets (years)	10.0	10.1	9.5
Cushion ratio (x)	9.9	8.2	5.3
Days cash on hand	145	111	86
Days in accounts receivable	50.9	51.5	52.9
Cash flow/total liabilities (%)	17.8	14.1	12.8
Unrestricted cash/long-term debt (%)	85.4	80.4	63.6
Long-term debt/capitalization (%)	37.0	40.7	45.0
Payment period (days)	58.4	56.2	58.9

Note: All figures as of June 20, 2005. Medians for 2005 are based on 2004 audited financial statements and 93% of rated credits.

Source: Standard & Poor's. 2005. *U.S. Not-for-Profit Health Care 2005 Median Ratios*. New York: Standard & Poor's, July. Used with permission.

2. *Decline in financial performance*: Weaker financial performance, either over a period of time or suddenly

3. *Erosion of market share*: The absence of a competitive strategy or the inability to compete with hospitals that are merging or affiliating

4. *Poor balance sheet management*: The failure to increase liquidity or a decline in liquidity, even if cash flow generation improves

5. *Subordination of existing bond security with a debt instrument that has greater or increased security features*: The pledging of enhanced security to other creditors, or the structural subordination of bondholders to other creditors who have direct access to the hospital's assets or cash flow

The following factors contribute to rapid and frequent rating downgrades:

- rapid depletion of cash, resulting in extremely low liquidity levels;

TABLE 2-4. Fitch Ratings: Nonprofit Hospital and Health Care System Medians, 2004

	Median	'AA'	'A'	'BBB'	Below 'BBB'
Sample size	220	37	95	63	25
Total operating revenue ($ mil)	313.3	1,434.4	302.8	153.9	138.6
Days cash on hand	157.8	232.3	177.2	117.5	49.3
Days in accounts receivable	51.5	51.9	51.4	51.3	51.0
Cushion ratio (x)	11.4	20.1	13.4	8.9	3.0
Days in current liablilities	64.5	66.3	61.5	63.7	69.2
Cash to debt (%)	99.4	152.5	109.8	82.1	32.8
Operating margin (%)	2.1	3.5	2.5	1.0	(1.8)
Excess margin (%)	3.7	5.9	4.2	2.4	(0.1)
EBITDA margin (%)	10.8	12.6	11.3	9.1	5.8
Cash flow margin	9.2	10.5	10.3	8.4	3.6
Investment income as % of excess income	35.0	42.0	37.4	34.3	18.8
Personnel costs as % of total operating revenue	51.6	51.2	50.2	52.5	55.7
Bad debt expense as % of total operating revenue	5.7	4.7	6.3	5.2	7.1
EBITDA debt service coverage (x)	3.3	4.8	3.5	2.8	1.6
CFFOBI debt service coverage (x)	3.3	4.3	3.6	2.7	1.6
CFFOBI debt service coverage less capital expenditures (x)	0.9	1.3	1.1	0.6	0.7
Maximum annual debt service as % of revenues	3.4	2.9	3.4	3.6	4.2
Debt to EBITDA (x)	3.7	2.9	3.5	4.1	5.2
Debt to free cash flow (x)	4.7	6.8	4.7	1.3	6.6
Debt to capitalization (%)	42.3	34.8	39.0	47.3	75.1
Average age of plant (years)	9.8	9.4	9.9	9.3	13.1
Capital expenditures as % of depreciation expense	133.3	153.8	138.8	128.3	101.4
Capital expenditures as % of EBITDA	66.7	66.3	64.0	70.5	44.8
Capital expenditures as % of total revenue	7.0	8.0	7.3	6.3	4.3

EBITDA–Earnings before interest, taxes, depreciation, and amortization. CFFOBI–Cash flow from operations before interest.

Source: Fitch Ratings, Inc. 2005. *2005 Median Ratios for Nonprofit Hospitals and Health Care Systems*. New York: Fitch Ratings, August. Used with permission.

- the heavy use of bank lines of credit or demand notes to meet immediate working capital needs, thereby increasing the debt burden;
- financial restatements of historical performance, resulting in lower-than-reported earnings; and
- management issues, such as the lack of communication or disclosure to the agency regarding decisions that may jeopardize debt security; ongoing turnover in senior management that results in multiple restatements of performance; or fraud or embezzlement.

Healthcare leaders should be familiar with industrywide trends related to credit rating upgrades and downgrades. The rate of bond downgrades by each of the three rating agencies significantly outpaced upgrades between 1998 and 2003 and slowed a bit in 2004. For the first time in many years, the proportion of upgrades exceeded downgrades by two of the three agencies in 2005.

Conducting a Financial Credit Analysis

A financial credit analysis allows an organization to compare its recent financial performance to relevant national standards that serve as a benchmark. Organizations typically use key indicators from S&P, Fitch Ratings, or Moody's for similarly rated organizations to construct the necessary data chart. These indicators include revenue, income, cash, and debt figures as well as profitability, debt, and liquidity ratios.

Table 2-5 provides a financial credit analysis chart for a sample "A" rated organization, Community Hospital. An analysis of the data enables the organization to draw conclusions or make key observations about relative performance. Observations about Community Hospital appear as Sidebar 2-5.

Corporate Finance–Based Strategies for Credit Fitness

Darwin's theory of evolution challenges healthcare leaders to ensure fitness for survival. Fitness standards are customary in the corporate world. The use of best practice corporate finance by the nation's not-for-profit healthcare organizations will play an important role in further strengthening an organization's ability to adapt to changing market and regulatory conditions.

TABLE 2-5. Financial Credit Analysis Highlights for Community Hospital (in Millions of Dollars)

Ratio/Statistic	S&P's "A"	Moody's "A"	Fitch "A"	Fiscal Year Ending June 30, Annualized 2002	2003	2004	2005
Net patient service revenue	$207,275	$274,330	—	$206,422	$216,888	$234,643	$238,655
Operating income	—	$6,724	—	$6,430	($1,118)	$1,180	$1,376
Net income	—	$14,785	—	($9,609)	$233	$5,322	$10,006
Cash flow (net income plus depreciation)	—	$31,607	—	$2,285	$11,540	$16,927	$21,087
Unrestricted cash	—	$118,246	—	$97,975	$121,300	$101,705	$111,527
Long-term debt	—	$120,109	—	$98,310	$99,160	$107,248	$110,513
Capital expenditures	—	$28,917	—	$6,880	$12,886	$16,303	$14,002
Profitability							
Operating margin	2.3%	2.2%	1.9%	2.9%	(0.5%)	0.5%	0.6%
Excess margin	3.1%	4.5%	2.9%	(4.7%)	0.1%	2.1%	3.9%
Operating EBIDA margin	9.1%	9.5%	8.2%	11.0%	7.0%	7.5%	7.4%
Debt Position							
Maximum annual debt Service coverage (x)	3.4	4.1	3.6	1.0	1.5	2.0	2.4
Debt to capitalization	36.5%	39.8%	40.7%	39.7%	38.9%	37.8%	37.2%
Liquidity							
Cash to debt	103.4%	101.9%	98.4%	91.2%	122.3%	94.8%	100.9%
Days cash on hand	167.0	155.2	170.9	177.6	203.3	160.6	172.3
Days in A/R, net	54.5	54.6	54.2	77.5	70.0	58.4	59.5
Other							
Average age of plant	9.1	9.2	9.3	12.9	6.8	7.5	8.9
Capital expenditure to operating revenue	—	—	—	3.1%	5.7%	6.7%	5.6%
Capital ratio	—	—	—	57.8%	114.0%	140.5%	126.4%
Compensation ratio	52.1%	—	50.8%	52.5%	52.0%	51.3%	52.1%

Notes: S&P's, Moody's, and Fitch Ratings data represent 2004 medians; compensation ratio is defined as salaries, wages, and benefits/total operating revenues. A/R=accounts receivable.

Source: Kaufman, Hall & Associates, Inc. Used with permission.

SIDEBAR 2-5. Creditworthiness Comments for Community Hospital

Revenue and Cost
- Community Hospital's net patient revenues are consistent in size with the "A" category medians.
- Net patient revenues grew by 8.2 percent from fiscal year 2003 to fiscal year 2004. Budget 2005 growth is projected to slow to approximately 1.7 percent. Relative to anticipated expense growth, this decelerating revenue growth can be a negative credit attribute.

Profitability and Cash Flow
- Community Hospital's profitability indicators improved from 2003 to 2004 but fell short of "A" rated levels. Budget 2005 profitability is projected to improve over previous years, but operating margin and earnings before interest, taxes, depreciation, and amortization (EBITDA) margin remain below "A" rated levels.
- Community Hospital's ability to continue to generate annual cash flow at levels equal to or better than 2004 will be vital to support strategic capital investment requirements. Budgeted cash flow in 2005 is projected to increase considerably, from $16.9 million to $21.1 million.

Debt Position
- Community Hospital has 2005 outstanding debt of $110.5 million, resulting in debt service coverage levels well below "A" rated medians.
- Debt to capitalization has come down from its 2002 peak level of 39.7 percent and continues to trend lower (it is projected to be 37.2 percent for 2005) as profitability continues and ongoing principal payments are made.

Liquidity
- Community Hospital's cash position eroded somewhat from 2002 to 2004, but it is forecast to improve significantly from 160.6 days in 2004 to 172.3 days in 2005.
- Relative to its debt load, as measured by the cash-to-debt ratio, Community Hospital's cash position is consistent with "A" rated medians.
- Maintenance of liquidity strength will be key to Community Hospital's ability to optimally access capital over both the short term and the long term.

Overall Credit-Related Recommendations
- Community Hospital should incorporate at least "A" median credit ratios into its periodic financial reporting to ensure ongoing awareness of the broad requirements to maintain access to capital.

Continued

SIDEBAR 2-5. (continued)

- Community Hospital must focus on maintaining the strength of its balance sheet and reversing the historical trends in its liquidity. It must focus on the following key areas of performance to support its long-term strategic plan and maintain access to external capital:
  — Maintain consistent, strong operating performance as measured by both the operating margin and operating EBIDA margin.
  — Manage cash flow to ensure ongoing retention and growth of cash reserves. This will entail strategic control of capital expenditures both with regard to total amounts and type of investment.

Source: Kaufman, Hall & Associates, Inc. Used with permission.

Hence, the first strategy is to act like GE.

But what does acting like GE really mean? Organizations will be required to apply the basic principles of corporate finance by asking and answering on a regular basis the essential questions outlined in Concept Three. Answering these questions requires linking strategic and financial issues.

The second strategy is to keep a close eye on the balance sheet. This is the organization's financial backbone. It indicates how leveraged the organization is and the liquidity available to buffer pressures on operating profits due to declining reimbursement. Income statements can fluctuate dramatically on a month-by-month basis, but the balance sheet must remain steady and on target (Wareham 2001).

Given the favorable low-interest-rate environment in recent years, many not-for-profit healthcare organizations have been turning to the debt market to fund an increasing number of major strategic initiatives. Taking on debt generally brings more risk, which at a certain level can stress the income statement, the balance sheet, and the organization's bond credit rating. Organizations operating according to corporate finance principles will not inappropriately deplete cash or incur debt beyond capacity. Lowering credit will increase debt capacity in the short run, but not in the long run. The long-term consequences of increased capital investment that degrades credit position are significant and lasting. History has demonstrated that balance sheet and rating declines are extremely difficult to reverse (Kaufman 2003 and 2004).

Some experts suggest that both the rating agencies and institutional bond buyers are currently applying balance sheet standards that are overly conservative. They argue that, given the very significant strategic investments that healthcare organizations need to make, some organizations (particularly those with "A"-category bond ratings) would be better served by spending down cash, borrowing at a higher level, and accepting the resulting lowered ("BBB") bond rating. This is not good advice for the following eight reasons:

1. *Hospitals should maintain a healthy respect for the capital markets.* Deliberately reducing bond ratings to accommodate strategic investment demonstrates a certain naiveté relative to the capital markets. Such a strategy assumes that "BBB" credits will always have easy and unfettered access to both capital and market liquidity. This is a pretty aggressive assumption. Just because this has been true in the post–World War II economy doesn't mean such conditions will prevail indefinitely.

2. *Organizations need to protect long-term debt capacity.* Lowering credit in the short run will increase debt capacity. However, in the long run, lowering credit will lower ratings and lower financial performance will decrease debt capacity. Deteriorating capital capacity has been a major competitive obstruction for many hospitals during the past decade.

3. *Ratings are "sticky down."* Lowering credit to accommodate incremental strategic investment implies that this "more" aggressive financial strategy will eventually produce substantial financial returns that will cause ratings to bounce back up over some period of time. Past performance does not support this. As economists say, "Bond ratings are sticky down." Once ratings decline, they infrequently go back up, and, if they do go back up, they go back up slowly.

4. *Pursuing the credit strategy described earlier exposes an individual hospital to significant additional credit risk.* Some questions are appropriate: How much liquidity will your organization need to compete long term? If you deliberately go below that level of liquidity to support current strategic investment, do you have a plan to replace lost liquidity? Will you ever recover lost liquidity?

5. *Hospitals must ensure continued community trust.* How does such a strategy relate to the fiduciary responsibility of your board and your management team? State attorneys general around the country have recently advocated a very conservative definition of the notion of "community

trust" and have clearly designated the not-for-profit hospital as a "community asset." How does the deliberate conversion of liquidity to strategy, given risky business conditions, jive with the preservation of the hospital as a community trust?

6. *Investment performance may not stay as it is.* How will a deliberate reduction in liquidity relate to your hospital's investment portfolio? What if stock market averages dropped 1,000 points at the same time you were converting cash to facilities and equipment? Would such a combination of events materially weaken your balance sheet or, perhaps, even threaten the solvency of your hospital?

7. *Hospitals need cash.* One observation critical to the credit discussion is the fact that for-profit providers keep very little cash on hand, especially compared to the not-for-profits. This observation ignores the fact that for-profits finance ongoing capital investment through equity, debt, and operating cash flow. The financing platform of the not-for-profits is entirely dependent on operating cash flow and debt. This is no small difference, and it places much greater emphasis on the quality of not-for-profit balance sheets.

8. *Hospitals should consider the impact on the industry's credit platform.* What is actually being suggested? Isn't hospital credit already deteriorating? The answer is, "absolutely." From 1988 through 2004, the rate of downgrades has significantly exceeded upgrades. Further deterioration of what has been until very recently a deteriorating credit platform should be avoided.

Debt capital remains available, but the bond and capital markets are increasing the requirements for access by healthcare organizations. Markets are expecting not-for-profit healthcare organizations to have the same kind of focus and attitude that publicly traded corporations maintain in dealing with Wall Street. This means real business plans, financial results that measure up to previous forecasts, a considerable attention to basics (such as expense control and revenue enhancement), consolidation and management of services, expert allocation of capital, and vigilant attention to reimbursement trends. Healthcare leaders must heed the financial assessments of rating agencies, bond insurers, and the institutional investor community.

Credit and creditworthiness are enduring concepts. Healthcare organizations that understand the importance of creditworthiness and maintain a strong credit position will do well in the future. Those that neither understand the factors underlying creditworthiness nor maintain a strong credit position are operating in uncertain circumstances. Their future is bleak.

References

Coile, R. 2002. *Futurescan 2002: A Forecast of Healthcare Trends 2002-2006.* Chicago: Health Administration Press.

Congressional Budget Office. "CBO's Current Budget Projections." [Online article; retrieved 3/2/06.] www.cbo.gov/budget/budproj.shtml.

Fitch Ratings. 2005a. *Healthcare Rating Actions for the Nine Months Ended Sept. 30, 2005.* New York: Fitch Ratings.

————. 2005b. *Rating Process for Nonprofit Healthcare Credits.* New York: Fitch Ratings.

Goldstein, L. 2005. "Integrating Strategy and Finance: Making the Case for Continuous Planning." Presented at the Kaufman Hall Financial Leadership Conference, Chicago, October 21, 2005.

Grube, M. E., and T. L. Wareham. 2005. "What is Your Game Plan? Advice from the Capital Markets." *Healthcare Financial Management* 59 (11): 63–75.

Healthcare Financial Management Association (HFMA). 2004. *How Are Hospitals Financing the Future: The Future of Capital Spending.* Westchester, IL: HFMA.

Kaufman, K. 2003. "Nine Observations on Credit Strategy for Not-for-Profit Hospitals." *Executive Insights* 1 (8): 1–3.

————. 2004. "Effective Financial Leadership: Walking the Walk vs. Talking the Talk." *Executive Insights* 2 (2): 1–3.

Moody's Investors Service. 2000. *An Updated Approach to Rating Not-for-Profit Healthcare Organizations.* New York: Moody's Investors Service.

———. 2002. *Not-for-Profit Healthcare Ratings*. New York: Moody's Investors Service.

———. 2004. *The Capital Spending Ratio (Special Comment)*. New York: Moody's Investors Service.

———. 2005a. *Not-for-Profit Healthcare: 2005 Outlook and Medians*. New York: Moody's Investors Service.

———. 2005b. *Indicators of Successful Management for Not-for-Profit Hospitals*. New York: Moody's Investors Service.

O'Neil, E. H. 2005. "The Workforce Challenge and Opportunity." In *Futurescan: Healthcare Trends and Implications 2005-2010*. Chicago: Health Administration Press.

Standard & Poor's. 2005a. *U.S. Not-For-Profit Healthcare 2005 Median Ratios*. New York: Standard & Poor's.

———. 2005b. *U.S. Not-for-Profit Healthcare Sector 2005 Mid-Year Outlook*. New York: Standard & Poor's.

———. n.d. *Not-for-Profit Healthcare: Inside the Rating Process*. New York: Standard & Poor's.

Wareham, T. L. 2001. "Strategies for Navigating the Healthcare Credit Market." *Healthcare Financial Management* 55 (4): 55.

CONCEPT THREE

Integrated Strategic and Financial Planning

To FIND THE Wizard in the Land of Oz, Dorothy and her friends simply followed the yellow brick road. One path. A fork here or there, but nothing too troublesome. One big decision—to proceed or not.

If only the healthcare world were as simple. It used to be. Hospitals were pretty much guaranteed a tomorrow through the retrospective cost-reimbursement system. Schooled in the social service aspect of healthcare delivery, administrators made decisions largely based on intuition, trial and error, and, if fortunate enough, experience.

Few healthcare executives need to be told that their world is a changed one, now characterized by continuous transformations. Rapidly developing communication and technological advances, increased competition, and a prospective reimbursement system have created an environment in which options, choices, and uncertainty abound. Experience, intuition, and trial and error no longer suffice as reliable executive decision-making tools. Why? The cost of making an error is just too high.

Overview of the Integrated Planning Process

Because survival is no longer a guaranteed option, wizard-seeking is a decidedly different process. The new process involves the methodical and thoughtful integration of strategy and finance through qualitative and quantitative thinking. Key to an organization's survival and success, the strategic and financial planning process is a continuous one. It includes identifying and selecting the strategies necessary to achieve the organization's purposes, ensuring the viability of such strategies through solid financial planning, and then directly and aggressively supporting selected strategies with the needed capital.

Most organizations have multiple purposes, and few organizations have sufficient capital capacity to meet their comprehensive strategic capital requirements. Policies, procedures, methods, and "rules of the road" must guide the integrated planning process to achieve the stated purpose(s) within the constraints of financial capability.

Corporate finance provides the navigational discipline used to answer the two key questions of strategic financial planning: What investments should be made? How should the investments be paid for? (Myers and Brealy 2003) As mentioned in Concept One, the organizing principle throughout the corporate finance–based process is as follows:

Financial performance must be sufficient to meet the cash flow requirements of the strategic plan and, at the same time, maintain or improve the financial integrity of the organization within an appropriate credit and risk context.

In some organizations, the planning process involves a strategic plan that is linked to a financial plan; in other organizations, the planning process results in one integrated plan. Either approach works if the plan provides the backbone for a healthcare organization, and

- links the organization's strategic mission and vision to measurable financial objectives;
- helps an organization determine whether strategies are financially possible given the organization's capital capacity;
- describes future financial risk in quantitative terms, considers alternative scenarios, and specifies sensible reactions to expected or unexpected changes; and
- enables the organization to react quickly and flexibly in a dynamic and complex marketplace.

The critical relationship between strategy and financial capability is illustrated in Figure 3-1. The organization's financial capability lies along the

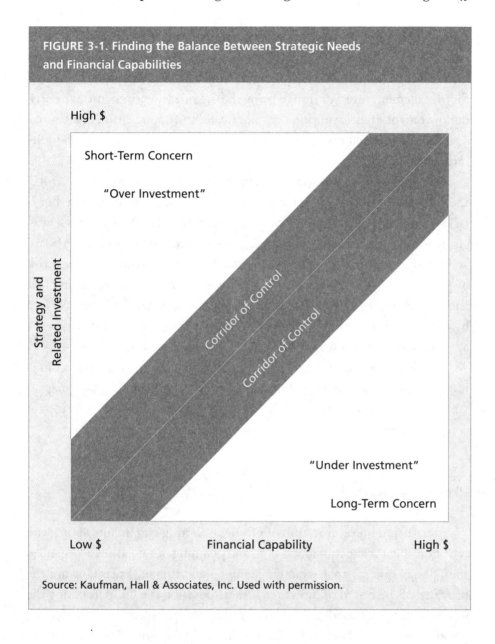

FIGURE 3-1. Finding the Balance Between Strategic Needs and Financial Capabilities

Source: Kaufman, Hall & Associates, Inc. Used with permission.

x axis; the organization's strategic financial requirements lie along the y axis. The "corridor of control" represents a balance between the two—in effect, an acceptable equilibrium situation. Over the long haul, every organization strives to achieve an appropriate balance between what it needs or wants to spend and what it actually can spend.

If an organization falls above the corridor of control in the area labeled "short-term concern," its financial need or strategic appetite exceeds its financial capability, and it is spending too much money. This signals the need for management intervention to bring the organization back into the corridor of control. If intervention does not occur, the organization could move so far to the left that no number of operating changes could bring about its return to equilibrium.

An organization whose position appears below the corridor of control in the area of long-term concern typically has a fair amount of money, but it lacks a strategic plan outlining how to grow and spend that money. Its strategic financial requirements may be fairly low because of a conservative board and management or other factors. Generally, such an organization is at risk of losing market share because it is not investing sufficient capital in plant and overall strategies while its competitors are doing so. Problems created by this approach manifest themselves more slowly than problems in the arena of short-term concerns.

The disciplined integration of strategic, financial, and capital planning, in an iterative and connected manner, results in an explicit road map to strategic and financial success, which keeps organizations in the corridor of control (Figure 3-2).

Planning leadership

The healthcare literature is full of often-conflicting statements about who is responsible for the mission, vision, and planning in a healthcare organization. Some indicate that strategic planning and financial planning are the province of the board of directors. Others describe the CEO as taking the lead, with the board of directors serving as a partner. Still others describe the planning as an equally shared responsibility. In reality, some boards establish mission, vision, and plans; others approve statements and plans developed by the CEO working with the board and senior executive colleagues.

We believe the board and senior management provide the *leadership* required for effective and integrated strategic and financial planning. Setting strategic direction and providing financial oversight are absolutely non-negotiable and integrally linked responsibilities. As stewards of their organizations, board members and senior leaders must understand the set

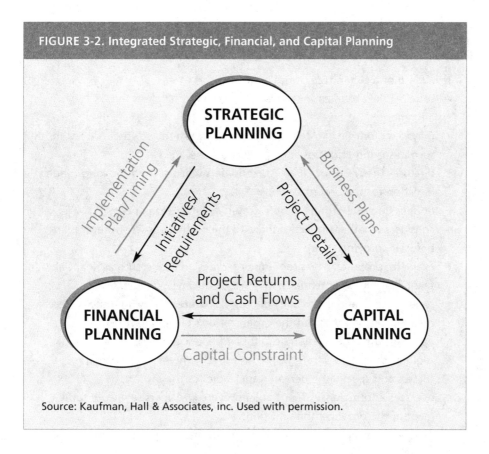

FIGURE 3-2. Integrated Strategic, Financial, and Capital Planning

Source: Kaufman, Hall & Associates, inc. Used with permission.

of strategies that ensure future competitiveness and the financial platform that conservatively supports such strategies.

In some organizations, the CEO is responsible for establishing a financial vision, which the board approves. The vision sets forth what the organization wishes to accomplish given its healthcare mission. It includes concrete financial goals and objectives. The CEO must have the financial training and experience necessary to establish the organization's long-term financial direction. For many, this means acquiring new skills and a working familiarity with analytical tools to remain at the helm. The CFO must be fully involved in the planning process. So too must the senior managers, middle managers, and clinical staff leaders who are responsible for making decisions and implementing plans.

Although the CEO and the CEO's management team are responsible for ground-level strategic and financial decisions, members of the board of directors must have a level of strategic and financial knowledge that enables them to participate in and support decisions (see Sidebar 3-1).

SIDEBAR 3-1. Strategic and Financial Responsibilities of the Board of Directors

The board or a committee of the board:
- requires the organization's strategic and financial plans to be in alignment;
- plays a major role in establishing the organization's strategic direction, such as setting priorities and approving the plan;
- discusses the needs of all key stakeholders when setting the long-range direction for the organization;
- defines how the organization's strategic plan is developed;
- considers whether projects adhere to the organization's strategic plan before approving them;
- evaluates proposed new programs or services on factors such as financial feasibility, market potential, and effect on quality and patient safety;
- reviews the financial feasibility of projects before approving those projects;
- rejects proposals that put the organization's mission at risk;
- approves the organization's capital and financial plans;
- requires that major strategic projects specify measurable criteria for success and specify the person responsible for the project;
- oversees a formal assessment at least every two years to ensure fulfill-ment of the organization's mission;
- reviews the organization's financial performance against plans at least quarterly; and
- demands corrective actions in response to underperformance on capital and financial plans.

Source: The Governance Institute. 2005. *Raising the Bar: Increased Accountability, Transparency, and Board Performance*. San Diego, CA: The Governance Institute, December. Used with permission.

Essentials of Strategic and Financial Planning

An organization's strategic plan or the strategy portion of an integrated plan focuses both on external market needs and how best to meet those needs with the organization's resources. Strategic planning comes before financial planning. It involves forecasting marketplace changes, such as demographics, payer mix, and reimbursement, and the effect such changes will have on the organization. Strategic planning proactively prepares the organization to use or create change to the organization's best advantage.

Mission and vision statements provide the foundation for a strategic plan. From these flow a set of critical goals or objectives that enable the organization to meet its mission. The goals must reflect a thorough assessment of an organization's market and strategic position, which provides the framework for understanding marketplace challenges and opportunities. Such understanding is critical to goal development.

Sidebar 3-2 outlines need-to-know information related to market and strategic positions. Key questions answered during the assessment process include the following:

- Which markets does the organization serve? What is the organization's market share? How has this changed over time?
- What are the current and projected future characteristics of the population and the local economy?
- What changes are anticipated in demand for healthcare services within the market? How will changes in demographics and emerging technologies affect future demand for hospital services?
- What is the organization's current service-delivery configuration and the condition of its physical assets?
- Who are the principal competitors? How are these competitors positioned, and what strategies are they pursuing? How will these strategies affect the organization's position?
- What key trends are occurring related to inpatient and outpatient service utilization?
- What are the organization's program/service strengths, weaknesses, and development opportunities?

Next, the plan defines the initiatives—the programs, services, or activities desired during the planning period. Utilization trends and demand projections based on the demographic and other market/strategic data collected by the organization enable leaders to identify future market size and opportunities for specific services lines within specific market areas. Projections must be based on assumptions that are plausible and defensible.

SIDEBAR 3-2. Need-to-Know Information Related to Market and Strategic Position

- *Patient origin*: Proportion of business from primary and secondary service area and/or specific geographic market clusters
- *Demographics*: Population, age, employment/unemployment rates, income (per capita and family)
- *Employers*: Large employers coming to or leaving the area, type of insurance provided
- *Market share*: Inpatient and outpatient (often difficult to obtain), by service line
- *Hospital/nonhospital competitors*: overall, by service line, nontraditional competition from physicians, diagnostic facilities, competitive strategies (niche versus full service)
- *Payer mix*: Medicare/Medicaid, commercial insurers, self-payers, provider/insurer dynamic (leverage? profitability of payers?), terms of private insurance and managed care contracts, incentives offered by insurers (quality measures), proportion of bad debt and charity care
- *Business, program, and service mix*: Unique niches, overall balance, performance and profitability by service line, secondary/tertiary/quaternary services
- *Physician staff*: Age, primary/specialty mix, proportion of revenue by specialty/physician, quality of relationships in referral base, loyalty, satisfaction, employment model, recruitment, dependence on one service
- *Employees*: Nurse and other employee retention strategies, turnover
- *Utilization/case mix*: Growth of good utilization/case mix (paying; high acuity) or bad utilization (nonpaying; low acuity), demand projections
- *Competitive cost/charge position*: Adjusted for outpatient volumes and case mix complexity, recent rate increases
- *Consumer preferences/opinions*: Survey information, as available

Source: Kaufman, Hall & Associates, Inc. Used with permission.

Market strength and competitive differentiation are critical to sustained competitive financial performance. An organization that does not currently maintain a strong position or is not clearly differentiated from its competitors should ensure that its integrated strategic and financial plan outlines a

---

SIDEBAR 3-3. Elements of Integrated Strategy and Finance

- A mission and vision statement
- An analysis of the organization's market and strategic position
- Identification of initiatives that will provide market strength and competitive differentiation
- Credible utilization and financial projections and assumptions
- Sensitivity analyses for key variables
- Financial planning for necessary resources
- Action plans, indicators and targets, and accountabilities
- A performance evaluation process

Source: Kaufman, Hall & Associates, Inc. Used with permission.

---

path to get there in the future (Grube and Wareham 2005). Sidebar 3-3 describes elements of integrated strategy and finance.

The financial plan or the financial planning portion of an integrated plan assesses the feasibility of identified strategies. A financial plan has a long time horizon—most commonly five years. It quantitatively identifies the profitability and liquidity requirements of the organization's strategic initiatives and addresses the issues of funding and financing required to meet such objectives. Multiyear financial planning is not an optional activity. To capital market players who rate and insure healthcare debt, the absence of multiyear financial planning discredits an organization's strategy. Credit position and capital access are at risk.

Simulation or sensitivity analysis, often called Monte Carlo simulation, helps healthcare leaders address the risks created by the simultaneous interaction of multiple strategic and financial plan elements, such as utilization projections, impact of competitive initiatives, and targeted productivity improvements. Best practice integrated planning includes such analyses to identify and gain insight into the key variables that could interact positively or negatively to affect the organization's competitive financial performance.

For example, to evaluate the desirability and feasibility of a major capital investment at one of its facilities, one health system used sensitivity analysis to review market, market share, demographic, utilization, expense, payment, and productivity projections. This enabled the organization to assess the major risks associated with key assumptions and potential strategic responses from competitors. The organization identified risks as follows:

- a 50 percent reduction of outpatient business due to physician joint venture initiatives;
- loss of 30 percent of volume resulting from the sale of a competing hospital and change in physician loyalty;
- increased population growth and need for additional investment to support higher volumes;
- failure to achieve planned productivity increases;
- increased insurance expense and inflation assumptions about utility expenses; and
- limited increases in Medicare and Blue Cross reimbursement rates.

Based on the analysis, the organization revised its baseline financial plan to factor in potentially reduced financial performance. The analysis reduced the risk of overstating the organization's financial capability, which, in turn, could have resulted in its approval of a higher level of capital spending than feasible for the organization.

The multiyear financial plan supports the strategic plan by answering seven critical questions:

1. What are the organization's strategic capital requirements?
2. How much cash should the organization have on hand?
3. How much debt can the organization afford?
4. What short-term and long-term profitability targets are necessary to resolve any shortfalls?
5. What level of operating change is required to meet the profitability targets?
6. Where will the capital be obtained in the short term and the long term?
7. What transactions are required to obtain the necessary capital?

A sophisticated healthcare financial plan includes the following:

- *Financial projections*: Developed from accurate, well-maintained databases, these are capable of interactive, real-time analysis.
- *Financial goals*: These are flexible and easy to recalculate to allow for changes in the marketplace and strategic investment requirements.
- *Capital expenditure requirements*: Covering a five-year period, these include hard-dollar (projects and technology) and soft-dollar (investments in physician networks and other integration initiatives) requirements.
- *Debt capacity and cash requirements*: These provide the "sources" side of the financial planning equation.
- *An analysis of capital position*: This compares the uses and sources of funds to identify any capital surplus or shortfall.
- *Profitability calculations*. These indicate the level of profitability that will close the capital shortfall and stabilize the organization.

Each portion of the plan is critical to obtaining the whole picture of an organization's financial health.

Conducting a credit analysis

The financial assessment begins with a credit analysis, which allows the organization to compare its recent financial performance to relevant national standards. It provides key indicators of financial strength and weakness and a benchmark of past and current creditworthiness. Organizations generally compare key indicators with Fitch Ratings, Standard & Poor's, or Moody's ratings for other organizations in selected bond-rating categories. For example, a hospital with an "A–" bond rating from S&P would compare itself to other medical centers with an "A–" S&P rating. The agencies publish rating data for not-for-profit hospitals and health systems on an annual basis.

Table 2-5 (see Concept Two) provides statistics and ratios for freestanding hospitals and single-state healthcare systems in 2004 and comparative data from a sample Community Hospital. Key observations drawn based on the comparison with national data appear as Sidebar 2-5 (see Concept Two). A full description of how to analyze your organization's creditworthiness also appears in Concept Two. This step is critical to the success of future strategic and financial planning.

Determining sources and uses of cash

The next step in the process is to define the financial and capital requirements necessary to ensure the organization's creditworthiness (i.e., profitability). This involves basic algebra. Uses of capital or the capital requirements appear on the left side of the equation. They include

- estimated capital requirements,
- funding required to maintain minimum cash position, and
- principal payments on debt.

Sources of capital appear on the right side of the equation. They include

- unrestricted cash and
- net available debt capacity.

The solution variable is the level of profitability necessary to balance the
uses/sources equation.

The journey to Oz begins with a single step, involving a reliable definition of financial requirements in year one (see Sidebar 3-4). Subsequent years
must be as carefully defined so that the organization can reach its longer-
term goals and objectives.

Capital uses

To solve the financial planning equation, leaders start by identifying the first
variable (capital requirements) on the left side of the algebraic equation. To
remain competitive, organizations must establish an appropriate level of
investment in their facilities and clinical programs. The organization's current
strategic capital requirements should be outlined and based on objectives
identified for the organization for each of the plan years. Competitive information obtained through national rating services (see age of plant information, for example, in tables 2-2 through 2-4 in Concept Two) can be useful for
purposes of comparison. Armed with information obtained through the
strategic planning process, the organization can develop a chart outlining capital expenditure requirements for the plan period.

SIDEBAR 3-4. Calculating Annual Financial Requirements

An organization's annual financial requirements can be calculated as follows:

	(1)	Annual capital expenditures
+	(2)	Changes in working capital
+	(3)	Actual principal payments
+	(4)	Incremental expansion of debt capacity
+	(5)	Increases in cash on the balance sheet
=	(6)	Total annual financial requirement

The first three requirements enable an organization to maintain survival-level financial performance. The fourth and fifth requirements enable an organization to perform competitively. Increased cash allows healthcare organizations to respond to the changing healthcare environment and preserve creditworthiness.

Source: Kaufman, Hall & Associates, Inc. Used with permission.

Next, the organization must determine its total capital shortfall. Capital shortfall is the summation of capital uses less the summation of capital sources.

Other capital requirements or uses appearing on the left side of the financial planning equation include the funding required to maintain a minimum cash position and principal payments on debt through the plan period.

Principal payments on debt can be determined based on the existing amortization schedules. The amount of minimum cash reserves is a major issue for many healthcare organizations. How much cash is enough cash? How much is needed to compete in a rapidly changing healthcare environment? Again, key competitive data from credit agencies can provide a starting place. One method of determining the minimum level of cash reserves is to use a days-cash-on-hand target. Another method uses the cushion ratio (cash and marketable securities plus board-designated funds divided by annual debt service). Competitive information on cash on hand and cushion ratios can be found in rating agency data (see tables 2-2 through 2-4 in Concept Two).

The target requirement for cash reserves can be calculated once an organization has determined the five-year projected cash operating expenses for the plan period. This figure is obtained by dividing the fifth-year cash operating expenses by 365 days to obtain a per-day cash requirement. Multiply this per-day requirement by the target days cash on hand of a similarly rated organization (obtained from agency data such as tables 2-2 through 2-4 in Concept Two). This yields the organization's target requirement for cash reserves.

Capital sources

Capital sources include unrestricted cash, net available debt capacity, and any other sources such as bond-related construction funds. The current-year figure for unrestricted cash should be the first capital source listed on the right side of the financial planning equation.

Debt capacity

This is the amount of debt an organization is capable of supporting within a particular credit-rating profile. This figure must expand each year if the organization wants to remain financially competitive. The ability to incur additional debt makes the organization more responsive to its market and more resilient to expected and unexpected changes.

For example, a hospital with a debt capacity of $50 million and outstanding debt of $40 million has a net debt capacity of $10 million. If the hospital's strategy calls for spending $20 million to build ambulatory clinics in year five of the plan, the financial plan should describe the incremental amount of debt capacity that must be added to the balance sheet every year to raise the extra $10 million for the purchases.

To determine debt capacity, organizations can use five approaches based on credit ratios:

1. Debt service coverage, which focuses on the relationship between current profitability and maximum annual debt service
2. Debt to cash flow, which focuses on the relationship of debt to the sum of total profits plus depreciation and amortization

3. Cash to debt, which focuses on the relationship between liquidity and debt
4. Debt service to revenue, which focuses on the relationship of maximum annual debt service to total operating revenue and
5. Debt to capitalization, which focuses on the relationship between debt and total capitalization

Table 3-1 provides approaches to calculating debt capacity. The calculations result in different debt capacities, so organizations will want to apply weightings to reflect the perceived importance of each approach. Generally, the debt service coverage, debt-to-cash flow, and cash-to-debt approaches are weighted higher than the debt-to-capitalization approach.

For example, the organization described in the case example later in this chapter calculated net available debt capacity as follows.

First, determine the cash flow available for debt service in the current year ($22.8 million in 2002, see Figure 3-6). Next, obtain from agency rating data the ratio for target debt service coverage of similarly rated organizations (3.7x). Divide the cash flow available for debt service by the ratio to determine a maximum annual debt service allowable figure ($22.8 million divided by 3.7x, which translates to a current debt capacity of $85 million, given current interest rates). Compare this figure to existing maximum annual debt service. The difference between the two will be net available debt capacity. Existing debt at the organization profiled in the case example is $57.6 million and, as a result, current available debt capacity is 27.4 million ($85 million minus $57.6 million).

Solving the financial equation

A capital position analysis integrates the left and right sides of the financial planning equation. This analysis compares the uses and sources of funds and calculates the expected capital shortfall or, in a very unusual circumstance, a capital surplus. Total capital requirements or uses for the organization in the case example are $256.3 million. Total capital sources are $162.8 million. The estimated five-year capital shortfall is $93.5 million. Figure 3-7 demonstrates a capital position analysis.

TABLE 3-1. Aproaches to Calculating Debt Capacity (in Millions of Dollars)

Ratio	Key Target	Indicated Capacity	Weighting
Debt service coverage	3.0x	$62.3	45%
Excess of revenue over expenses + Interest +			
Depreciation + Amortization/MADS			
Debt to cash flow	4.0x	60.3	15%
Long-term debt + Short-term debt/Excess of			
revenue over expenses + Depreciation +			
Amortization			
Cash to debt	100%	38.3	15%
Cash and marketable securities + Board-			
designated funds / Long-term debt +			
Short-term debt			
Debt service to revenue	4.0%	49.1	15%
Maximum annual debt service /			
Total operating revenue			
Debt to capitalization	50%	68.0	10%
Long-term debt (less current portion)/			
Long-term debt (less current portion) +			
Unrestricted net assets			
Weighted capacity		$57.0	

Note: Certain ratio definitions vary a bit by rating agency.

Source: Kaufman, Hall & Associates, Inc. Used with permission.

The challenge at this point is to determine the level of cash flow needed to balance the financial equation. In this case example, Figure 3-8 illustrates the example organization's operating cash flow requirements for the five-year plan period at differing levels of capital investment. If this organization wants to invest $75.5 million during the plan period, it must generate an average annual cash flow of $18.6 million to close the cash shortfall.

This organization must now ask and answer a key question: "Is that level of cash flow attainable?" In other words, does the projected financial performance of the system under business-as-usual operating assumptions in fact support a $75.5 million capital investment over five years? If the answer to this question is yes, then the strategies on which the plan is based are financially feasible given the organization's capabilities. The organization can confidently proceed with its intended strategy.

If the answer to the question is no, the organization must ask another key question: "Could we make changes in our operations and strategies to achieve that level of profitability?" To close the capital shortfall and meet profitability targets, this organization would need to reduce capital spending, improve market share and revenues, or reduce operating costs. Without such changes, the organization's strategic plan would not be viable. New strategies with new financial projections would be required.

Figure 3-8 indicates that that level of cash flow is attainable but that projected annual cash flow will not support higher levels of spending.

Ensuring reasonable goals

To ensure realistic projections, goals must be measurable and objective. Realistic profitability goals reflect the level of cash flow needed to meet all of the organization's financial requirements outlined in its strategic plan. The key question is, "Is it reasonable to expect this organization to operate at the projected level of profitability?" Financial forecasts and target and sensitivity analyses are helpful tools for testing the assumptions behind the financial plan for the organization's financial performance. These tools involve using best practice forecasting techniques by identifying risk points and developing "what if" scenarios for key operating indicators. For example, sensitivity analyses would explore the financial implications of "what if hospital inpatient volume or hospital productivity decreased?" or "what if salary inflation rates were higher than projected?"

Using competitive benchmarks to test the realism of profitability goals is not recommended. Although one might find it tempting to focus on the operating margin experienced by similarly rated hospitals, this number would not be an appropriate profitability goal for an organization requiring considerable capital for a new facility, for example. This organization would require a much higher goal. If the organization in the case example aims for the 1.2 percent operating margin achieved by "A" rated organizations, for example, it will fall far short of meeting its capital needs. Financial goals should be developed from the results of the financial plan. Benchmarking in this case puts the cart before the horse, requiring the development of a financial plan based on established goals.

Enhancing the effective implementation of the plan

Implementation of the plan can be enhanced by ensuring organizationwide input into the plan's development and providing the opportunity and enough information for every member of the organization to participate in achieving the plan's goals and objectives. Key constituencies—including management, the board, clinical staff, middle managers, the community, and lenders—must understand the goals. Carefully prepared materials presenting organizational objectives and describing how the leadership plans to achieve them should be made available to key constituencies. Understanding provides an organizationwide sense of ownership in financial direction.

A well-developed and executed financial plan is key to an organization's survival and success in the current healthcare environment. In the Wizard of Oz, Dorothy wakes up "in full color" and exclaims, "Toto, I've got a feeling we're not in Kansas anymore." It is indeed a different healthcare world.

Case Example: Planning in Practice

This example describes an organization's implementation of the corporate best practice integrated planning process to ensure continued creditworthiness and solid financial performance. Although the process occurred more than five years ago in the example organization, it remains equally valid today as an illustration of the planning and analysis principles presented in Concept Two and Concept Three. Although the organization's name is fictitious, the information presented is real.

The organization at a glance

Community Hospital Healthcare System (CHHS) is a not-for-profit organization located in the suburbs of a major metropolitan area. Its 290-bed flagship hospital is noted for excellence in numerous clinical areas. Drawing patients from a service area of nearly 1 million residents, the hospital enjoys a sizable 35 percent share of the region's highly competitive acute care market.

Like many other organizations in the 1990s, CHHS positioned itself as an integrated health system and market consolidator. That view of the organization has changed. Says the CEO, "We now recognize that we are, at heart, a hospital. We must ensure that our patients have a continuum of care, but we don't have to own the full range of service providers."

Financial history

CHHS had achieved strong financial results throughout its 60-year history. The organization's consistent "A1"/"A+" credit rating reflected this, as did the hospital's status as the most profitable facility in the state. Staff tenure was high, and turnover was consistently low. During the late 1990s, when many organizations were struggling, CHHS's performance was exceptionally strong. The organization accumulated large sums of cash during these years and outperformed its competitors through zealous cost management and what the new CEO calls "some real skill with the reimbursement system."

However, significant cost cutting, which was needed to sustain high profit levels, was eroding the strength of the hospital's core patient care areas. "If you're achieving profitability that significantly exceeds that experienced by competitors, you have to consider whether you're investing in those areas that are critical to the organization's long-term future," notes the CEO. In fact, the hospital's main campus was aging, undersized, and badly in need of improvement. At the same time, because education and training budgets and salary increases were cut to bare-bones levels, staff were becoming increasingly unhappy. Although capital flowed to endeavors such as physician practices and on-site outpatient centers, CHHS's core business was slowly being starved.

With nationwide healthcare staffing shortages in the late 1990s, CHHS's turnover and vacancy rates increased. Agency and temporary staff were hired to fill positions. "The financial bottom started falling out in 1999 and 2000, but a reimbursement windfall masked the signs and symptoms of the decline," notes the CEO.

A changing financial environment

In the fall of 2001, CHHS's new management team, which had been in place for no more than 60 days, found itself in an emerging financial crisis that required immediate attention. Key financial indicators revealed a significant and unexpected downturn. At the same time, the organization badly needed to proceed with Phase 1 capital expenditures. Approved in the late 1990s, these expenditures would help CHHS maintain its competitive position. Beyond Phase 1 expenditures, CHHS's board believed the hospital required an additional Phase 2 makeover that would cost $90 million. This capital would be used to construct an improved acute care campus and to provide new services, such as cardiac surgery, that promised increased revenues. Could CHHS afford the Phase 2 program? The organization faced a clear financial "fork in the road."

Implementing a best practice approach to financial planning

The CEO and management team put in place a best practice corporate financial planning process during the final months of 2001. This would help the board and the senior management team evaluate the feasibility of the Phase 2 capital plan and would link strategic, capital, and financial planning organizationwide.

Implementation of the best practice approach proceeded in an integrated fashion, enabling an aerial view of the organization's financial "forest" along with its component "trees." The key steps were as follows:

- Step 1: Understand credit
- Step 2: Understand capital
- Step 3: Understand liquidity
- Step 4: Understand debt capacity
- Step 5: Understand the capital position analysis
- Step 6: Understand cash flow targets
- Step 7: Retest the capital position analysis and cash flow targets to evaluate feasibility of increased capital expenditures

A summary of each step follows.

Step 1: Understand credit

The first step was to gain an understanding of the importance to the organization of effectively managing its credit position. A healthy "A1"/"A⁺" bond rating was one of CHHS's most important assets. Protecting the rating was imperative. A credit analysis, similar to one that would be performed by or for a rating agency, was conducted in January 2002. Median data from "A" rated organizations were included for comparison purposes.

The credit analysis (Figure 3-3) revealed a number of negative trends:

- *Operating and net income*: Operating and net income had declined significantly. Although net income was high in 2000 because of investment earnings from unrestricted cash, it declined dramatically when the stock market slid in 2001. Poor returns on investments, combined with poor operating results, were putting CHHS in a precarious financial position. For the first time, the operating margin was in the red in 2002.
- *Capital expenditures*: Due to deferral in earlier years, CHHS had committed to spending $41 million in 2002—its worst financial year in history.
- *Unrestricted cash*: Cash dropped between 2001 and 2002.
- *Long-term debt*: The organization's low level of debt would enable CHHS to borrow in the future. However, because the organization had not borrowed to pay for 2002 capital expenditures, it would have to use available cash to cover this expense. The organization's low debt-to-capitalization ratio reflected its funding of capital requirements through operating and investment income.

FIGURE 3-3. Credit Analysis

Ratio/Statistic	Moody's "A"	2000	2001	2002
Operating income ($000s)	—	8,920	5,464	(2,897)
Net income ($000s)	—	26,061	14,994	5,166
Capital expenditures ($000s)	—	11,467	14,844	41,771
Unrestricted cash ($000s)	—	148,404	151,681	142,168
Long-term debt ($000s)	—	62,931	61,266	57,695
Operating margin (%)	1.2	6.1	3.4	(1.8)
Excess margin (%)	3.7	16.0	8.9	3.0
Debt service coverage (x)	3.7	8.1	6.2	4.2
EBITDA margin (%)	—	16.5	13.2	9.0
Debt to capitalization (%)	36.5	24.6	23.6	21.7
Cushion ratio (x)	13.5	29.3	30.6	26.4
Days cash on hand	164.2	432.4	392.6	338.4
Compensation ratio (%)	—	44.5	44.8	47.4

Source: Kaufman, Hall & Associates, Inc. Used with permission.

As perhaps the key indicator of credit position in the not-for-profit health-care market, CHHS's days-cash-on-hand data provided the most revealing picture of the organization's financial performance. The organization maintained cash-on-hand balances two to three times higher than industry medians for similarly rated organizations. Higher cash balances tend to correlate to higher credit ratings. Balance sheet liquidity was supporting CHHS's whole credit profile and certainly its credit rating. When unrestricted cash declined in 2001 and 2002 and operating expenses increased significantly due to higher malpractice premiums and nursing agency costs (see increasing compensation ratio), days cash on hand started sliding. A decline of nearly 100 days occurred between 2000 and 2002. This increased the organization's credit risk.

Step 2: Understand capital

The next step was to answer the question, "How much money does CHHS need to spend to remain competitive and meet its strategic objectives?" The

FIGURE 3-4. Annual Capital Requirements: 2003–2007 (in 000s)						
	2003	**2004**	**2005**	**2006**	**2007**	**Total**
Capital requirements	$21,424	12,918	14,751	13,249	13,250	**$75,592**

Source: Kaufman, Hall & Associates, Inc. Used with permission.

CEO and the leadership team estimated baseline capital expenditures of $75 million for the forthcoming five-year period (Figure 3-4). This was the minimum amount of capital needed given continued less-than-acceptable financial performance. Phase 2 capital expenditures were not included. An accurate estimate of annual capital requirements was absolutely critical to the next steps in the financial planning process.

Step 3: Understand liquidity

The third step in implementing a best practice financial planning process was to understand liquidity or cash position. The goal was to answer the question, "How much cash should CHHS have?" The leadership team estimated annual and daily cash operating expenses in 2007 based on 2001 actuals and an inflationary factor. To maintain its "A1"/"A+" credit rating, CHHS wanted to keep its days cash on hand to no less than 300 days. This highlighted the critical need to focus on returning operating income to positive levels. The cash target for 2007 represented the product of the days-cash-on-hand target and per-day operating expenses (Figure 3-5).

The cash reserve analysis shed an entirely new light on the organization's cash position. In past years, board members questioned the need for high cash levels. The organization funded capital expenditures by drawing down cash reserves. The difference between the 2007 cash target and the 2002 unrestricted cash reserve made it apparent that CHHS needed a higher level of cash and certainly could not afford to spend its cash on budgeted capital expenditures. Doing so would threaten its credit rating.

FIGURE 3-5. Calculation of Minimum Cash Reserve (in 000s)	
	Minimum Target
Estimated 2007 cash operating expenses	$200,785
Estimated expenses per day	$550
Days-cash-on-hand target	300
2007 cash target	$165,029
2002 preliminary unrestricted cash reserve	**$142,168**
	(338 days cash)

Source: Kaufman, Hall & Associates, Inc. Used with permission.

Step 4: Understand debt capacity

The fourth step answered the question, "How much debt can the organization afford?" The most meaningful way for CHHS to estimate debt capacity was to take a look at the cash available to pay back debt. Figure 3-6 illustrates this approach.

If CHHS had wanted to borrow up to the maximum amount possible in 2000, its incremental net debt capacity was nearly $90 million. However, operating cash flow in the next two years would not have sustained that level of debt. Because borrowing would be required in the future, the organization needed to improve debt capacity through better operating results.

Step 5: Understand the capital position analysis

The fifth step answered the question, "What is the magnitude of the organization's capital shortfall (or surplus)?" By comparing capital uses and sources to identify the surplus or shortfall, the approach offers an integrated way of determining the capital required to balance the equation. Figure 3-7 clearly indicates that CHHS had insufficient cash flow to meet its ongoing financial requirements.

FIGURE 3-6. Incremental Debt Capacity (in 000s)

	2000	2001	2002
Cash flow analysis			
Revenues over expenses	$26,061	$14,994	$5,166
Interest	3,591	3,484	3,578
Depreciation	11,447	12,050	14,109
Income available for debt service	41,099	30,528	22,853
Expected debt service coverage (x)	3.7	3.7	3.7
Maximum debt service	11,108	8,251	6,177
Cash flow approach			
Estimated debt capacity	152,898	113,571	85,020
Existing long-term debt	62,931	61,266	57,695
Net debt capacity	89,967	52,305	27,325

Source: Kaufman, Hall & Associates, Inc. Used with permission.

Step 6: Understand cash flow targets

The sixth step answered the question, "What is the level of operating change required to meet the targets?" Figure 3-8 provides a look at the minimum required cash flow at various levels of capital expenditure. At the baseline expenditure level, CHHS could meet its cash flow needs. With increased capital expenditures of either $40 million or $90 million, the organization would need to achieve the cash flow levels experienced in 2000 and 2001.

Step 7: Retest the capital position analysis and cash flow targets to evaluate feasibility of increased capital expenditures

At this point, CHHS addressed the question of whether it could afford to spend the additional $90 million requested for a Phase 2 capital program. Retesting the capital position analysis and the cash flow targets would provide an accurate and dependable answer. Figure 3-9 depicts a re-forecasted

Figure 3-7. Capital Position Analysis (in 000s)

Uses		Sources	Without New Debt
Ongoing capital requirements	$75,592	Unrestricted cash 2002	$142,168
Principal payments (5 yrs)	10,450		
Target cash required (days cash on hand, 2007: 300)	165,029	Net debt capacity	0
Working capital	5,288	Other sources of cash	20,700
Total capital uses	**$256,359**	**Total capital sources**	**$162,868**
Total capital surplus (shortfall)			**($93,491)**

Source: Kaufman, Hall & Associates, Inc. Used with permission.

FIGURE 3-8. Cash Flow Targets (in 000s)

Capital Projects FY 2003-2007	Minimum Required Cash Flow*	
	Total Five Year	Average Annual
$75,592 (baseline)	$93,491	$18,698
$115,592 (baseline + $40M)	$133,491	$26,698
$165,592 (baseline + $90M)	$183,491	$36,698
Projected 2002 cash flow		**$19,237**
Actual 2001 cash flow		**$27,044**
Actual 2000 cash flow		**$37,508**

* Cash flow is defined as net income plus depreciation and amortization.
Source: Kaufman, Hall & Associates, Inc. Used with permission.

capital position analysis with the addition of $90 million of new capital spending under two scenarios. Without new debt, the capital shortfall would be $186 million; with new debt, the capital shortfall would be reduced by approximately $50 million.

FIGURE 3-9. Revised Capital Position Analysis: 2003–2007 (in 000s)

Uses		Sources	Without New Debt	With New Debt
Capital projects	$88,142	Unrestricted cash 2002	$142,168	$142,168
Ongoing requirements	75,592			
		Net debt capacity	0	50,000
Capital inventory uses	**163,734**	Less non-project proceeds	0	(1,000)
		Effective debt capacity	0	(49,000)
Principal payments (5 yrs)	13,216			
Total cash required (days cash on hand, 2007: 300)	167,396	Other sources of cash	20,700	20,700
Working capital	4,970			
Total capital uses	**$349,316**	**Total capital sources**	**$162,868**	**$211,868**
Total capital surplus (shortfall)			**($186,448)**	**($137,448)**

Source: Kaufman, Hall & Associates, Inc. Used with permission.

Next, CHHS revised its analysis of cash flow targets (Figure 3-10). Without new debt, the organization would have to ensure an average annual cash flow last achieved in 2000; with new debt, the required cash flow would need to be at the 2001 level. Under either scenario, the data made it clear that the larger capital expenditure was not sustainable at projected 2002 operating levels. Could the organization generate cash at levels achieved in 2000 or 2001? If not, the Phase 2 capital program should not be approved.

If CHHS had used a typical incremental decision-making process, the organization could have suffered permanent financial harm. Incremental decision making typically would have proceeded as follows:

- Incremental decision 1: Spend the additional $90 million.
- Incremental decision 2: Try to achieve $27 million in annual cash flow.
- Incremental decision 3: Because CHHS is nervous about the ability to achieve cash flow of $27 million, don't borrow additional money.

Whammo! An incremental process would have sunk the organization. Unable to achieve even $27 million in annual cash flow, CHHS would have needed an unreachable $37 million to cover the additional $90 million for the Phase 2 program. The program simply would not be affordable.

Lessons learned

Luckily, CHHS used an integrated approach to financial decision making that permitted an aerial view of the forest. The board and management team concluded that the organization could not afford the full Phase 2 capital program but needed to stick to the $75 million baseline capital budget until operating results improved. What else did they learn?

1. *Credit rating matters.* The organization's current rating was supported historically by an excellent cash position, strong profitability, and low levels of debt. Projected 2002 results would negatively affect both net income and days cash on hand. If these results persisted in future years, the organization's "A1"/"A+" rating would be downgraded.
2. *The actual amount of the capital plan matters.* Capital requirements ranged

FIGURE 3-10. Revised Cash Flow Targets (in 000s)

Capital Projects FY 2003-2007		Minimum Required Cash Flow*	
		Total Five Year	Average Annual
$163,734 (Revised baseline)	Without new debt	$186,448	$37,290
$163,734 (Revised baseline)	With new debt	137,448	27,490
Projected 2002 cash flow			19,237
Actual 2001 cash flow			27,044
Actual 2000 cash flow			37,508

* Cash flow is defined as net income plus depreciation and amortization.
Source: Kaufman, Hall & Associates, Inc. Used with permission.

between $75 million and $165 million. Spending beyond $75 million could not be supported by the organization's current operating performance.

3. *Restoring debt capacity to historical levels is essential.* Historical debt capacity was excellent. Current debt capacity was dramatically reduced because of declining operating results.

4. *The organization must not further increase the capital shortfall.* Assuming maintenance capital only, the capital shortfall was manageable. With the larger project, the capital shortfall (without additional debt) was insurmountable.

5. *The current cash flow target supported only maintenance capital, and expected cash flow in 2002 supported only baseline, maintenance capital.* Additional capital expenditure required greatly improved operating performance.

6. *Financial planning must be integrated with capital structure.* A decision to move forward with the $90 million Phase 2 plan required both operating improvement and $50 million of additional debt.

7. *Set a floor for and maintain at least the minimum days-cash-on-hand target.* The "A1"/"A+" bond rating was supported by the organization's strong cash position. Cash on hand must not fall beneath a floor of 300 days at least until the organization dramatically and permanently improved profitability.

Following are the organization's new financial goals and objectives:

- Increase cash flow to 2001 levels of $27 million.
- Bring debt capacity back to 2001 levels.
- Maintain cash on hand at 300 days.
- Borrow $50 million as soon as financial results support the "A1"/"A+" bond rating.

Says the CEO, "After completing the financial and credit analysis, we called a 'time-out' on the major expansion project. We're rethinking it in terms of our clinical priorities and the need to make it and other strategic initiatives more manageable. In the meantime, we're making some short-term investments in our operations, such as in the emergency department and patient care units, to ensure capacity needed in the community. These changes are being made to preserve our balance sheet within the context of a 'big picture' financial plan that is tied to our strategic plan."

Any erosion of the balance sheet will be carefully monitored. On a regular and ongoing basis, the management team will test and evaluate future course changes and their impact on the financial plan. Through use of a corporate finance-based approach to planning and analysis, CHHS is well on its way to improved financial performance.

A special note of thanks to CHHS's chief executive officer who helped "tell this story" in a way that would be helpful to other healthcare organizations.

References

The Governance Institute. 2005. *Raising the Bar: Increased Accountability, Transparency, and Board Performance*. San Diego, CA: The Governance Institute.

Grube, M. E., and T. L. Wareham. 2005. "What is Your Game Plan? Advice from the Capital Markets." *Healthcare Financial Management* 59 (11): 63–75.

Myers, S. C., and R. A. Brealy. 2003. *Principles of Corporate Finance*, 7th ed. Boston: McGraw-Hill/Irwin.

CONCEPT FOUR

Allocating Capital

Jason H. Sussman

IMAGINE TRYING TO play baseball without any rules. Three strikes don't make an out, so the neighborhood bully remains at the plate swinging away for hours. When he tires, whoever races to the plate first gets to hit next. Teams do not have a set number of players on the field, so team A has 18 people positioned between center and right field, and team B has only one player covering the whole outfield. Who will win this game? In fact, is this a game worth playing? Without a level playing field, wouldn't and shouldn't one team quit in disgust?

Overview of the Capital Allocation Process

An organization that has successfully implemented the strategic and financial planning process described in Concept Three has ensured that it has sufficient resources (i.e., capital) to support its strategic objectives. Now comes the equally important task of deciding how to deploy or allocate that capital. All sophisticated healthcare organizations have strategic and capital investment requirements that significantly exceed currently available capital capacity. Capital allocation involves determining whether any or all of the many potential capital projects or initiatives generated during the planning process make sense for the organization. It entails separating the wheat from the chaff on a level playing field that keeps all of the players in the game.

71

Why is capital allocation important? The long-term success of a healthcare organization is highly dependent on the capital investment decisions it makes today. Every decision either adds to or reduces the value of the overall operation. The cumulative effect of these incremental decisions determines the organization's future financial success. The most important financial decision made each year by senior management and ratified by the board is how much capital to spend and on what projects and initiatives the dollars will be spent.

Decisions must add to the organization's value—to its ability to generate capital for future projects, maintain or improve its creditworthiness, and accomplish its mission. For every investment that does not generate the expected revenue or value, the organization must seek other ways to obtain the cash flow and capital that should have been generated.

Revenue sources are harder and harder to find. In an environment of constrained reimbursement, scarce resources, and increased competition, the cost of making bad capital-investment decisions is both immediate and severe. The safety net provided in the past era by cost reimbursement and indemnity insurance no longer exists. Credit markets have tightened; the industry's operating cash flow is constantly challenged. To survive and succeed in the current environment, an organization's capital allocation process must be based on principles of corporate finance, involving rigorous and consistent application of proven quantitative techniques, as discussed later in the chapter.

Healthcare organizations often confuse capital allocation with the capital budgeting process. *Capital budgeting*, in fact, is just a small piece of the comprehensive corporate finance–based capital allocation process. It is the administrative process organizations use to spend capital that has been allocated. Capital budgeting often relates only to so-called routine capital items, such as minor replacements, that fall under the department manager's purview. It generates the detailed listing of purchases that will be made by departments during the next fiscal year. The capital budgeting process is administratively driven rather than analytically or strategically driven. Its success is measured by such criteria as "time required to complete" and "variance of proposed expenses from budget." Strategic financial concerns are seldom included among success indicators.

In contrast, the success of a *capital allocation* process is directly tied to the organization's strategic financial success. Available dollars are closely linked to the organization's long-term financial vision, and approved allocations create an overall portfolio that will generate an optimal return. Unlike the capital budgeting process, the capital allocation process comprehensively considers the short- and long-term implications of each potential investment within an overall portfolio of investments.

By nature, capital allocation involves politics and money. Because the process allocates capital, it also allocates influence and power within an organization. With so much at stake, the process must be led and supported by the CEO. If CEO leadership is not at the forefront, the organization naturally will use more informal, subjective approaches to allocation.

Traditional Approaches to Capital Allocation

Many not-for-profit healthcare organizations have historically approached capital allocation on a subjective basis, essentially ignoring quantitative analysis. They seem to assume that their core business can generate sufficient cash flow on an ongoing basis to support investment initiatives that may not have acceptable returns. Many organizations continue to allocate capital subjectively. The department, service, or unit that demands the most gets the most. This is a *political allocation approach*. The problem? Squeaky wheels with newly applied capital grease do not always bring the best returns.

Another approach is to allocate capital according to what was allocated the previous year. Under this type of *historical benchmark approach*, if a hospital's radiology department or one hospital in a multihospital system received $x million or x percent of the total capital dollars this year, it would expect to receive the same and maybe even an increased number of dollars or a similar share next year. The problem is that in today's turbulent healthcare environment, past performance may not be the best predictor of future results. For example, investing in physician practices, prevalent in the late 1990s, created significant losses rather than expected profitability.

Perhaps the most prevalent approach to capital allocation in healthcare is the *first come–first served approach*. In many organizations, specific projects are evaluated in a serial fashion as they arise throughout the calendar year. The critical problem is that, at the end of the fiscal year, no capital may be left to fund a project capable of bringing significant growth to the organization.

The *balanced scorecard approach* purports to evaluate both quantitative and qualitative management issues. Decision criteria include, for example, whether various new initiatives would meet community needs or increase physician satisfaction. Although worth considering during the decision-making process, such qualitative factors must be properly quantified. For example, if a proposed project is designed to meet the qualitative goal of enhancing physician satisfaction, the approach gives the project high marks in that particular criterion. No quantification is provided. Corporate finance–based capital allocation would force the analysis to go a step further and quantify the potential impact of increased satisfaction. Will the physicians increase their utilization of hospital services? If so, what revenue increases could be expected? Will ancillary usage be increased? If so, by what amount? Clearly, the answers to these questions will often be estimates. However, quantifying possible outcomes provides the organization with some measure of the investment's potential return.

An additional problem with the balanced scorecard approach is its formulaic use of multiple, weighted criteria that really does no more than codify the subjectivity of the group that established the weightings. For example, if there are ten criteria, one of which is the project's financial return, it is possible that only 10 percent of the decision weighting would be assigned to financial return. No organization can survive in the long run if it consistently pursues a series of investment decisions that are "strategically" driven to the detriment of the organization's financial position.

Finally, the *go-with-the-flow approach* to capital allocation involves no methodology and no articulated policy. The organization tries to fund whatever comes along, without the benefit of an evaluative process. The problem here is that not to decide is in fact to decide by default.

Characteristics and Benefits of a Best Practice Process

A best practice approach to capital allocation for healthcare organizations should be akin to the approach many *Fortune* 500 corporations use. That approach is based on a contemporary definition of capital, which extends beyond the traditional items such as property, plant, and equipment to embrace everything that appears on the cash flow statement. It includes such items as working capital funding for investment, start-up losses, joint venture investments, and all other items that take cash out of the organization.

Furthermore, the corporate approach includes the following key elements:

- link to a sound strategic financial plan;
- a solid business plan for each investment opportunity;
- standardized, one-batch project review;
- quantitative analysis using corporate finance–based techniques;
- data-driven and team-based decision making;
- coordinated calendar and planning cycles;
- clear definition of available capital;
- high level of governance, education, and communication; and
- process integrity through project monitoring and measurement.

A description of each follows.

Link to a sound strategic financial plan

Capital allocation must be based on a sound and integrated strategic financial plan. The plan must include good ideas worthy of investment. If the ideas articulated in the plan will not generate revenue, the management team should go back to the drawing board and identify ideas that will do so, find someone who can, or, if all else fails, get out of the business. A sound plan creates the framework to generate required capital capacity. Operating targets outlined in the plan and tied to the long-term strategy specify the amount of cash flow available each year to fund capital investments.

The capital allocation process must have clearly articulated objectives and principles. For example, a multihospital system might include in its written description of the capital allocation process two key principles covering the consolidation of capital available for investment and access to capital. The first principle states that all cash generated by all of the organizations within the system will be consolidated and will be available to meet all needs within the system. The second principle states that all organizations within the system have equal access to cash flow generated by system components.

Even though a facility may be losing money, it will be offered access to capital for an opportunity that is judged to represent potential for significant return. Such principles must be articulated and agreed to up front.

A solid business plan for each investment opportunity

To facilitate informed decision making, each investment opportunity must benefit from a thorough business plan, which describes the idea and its financial effect in significant detail. The business plan provides the basic documentation and analysis necessary for capital decisions. Components of a proper business plan appear as Sidebar 4-1.

Standardized, one-batch project review

The capital allocation process must include a specific, standardized project-review process that is applied consistently. Using standardized formats or templates for every project under consideration helps ensure true comparability. Rational and consistent evaluative guidelines and uniform decision criteria ensure unbiased decision making.

Not all proposed projects may warrant detailed financial analysis. Most organizations set a threshold for capital expenditures that will require detailed and centralized review. The threshold is based on the size and/or risk of the proposed investment. In the first year of implementing a best practice allocation process, the threshold should include 50 to 60 percent of total dollars to be spent, perhaps covering 20 to 30 projects. As the organizational process evolves and management grows more comfortable with it, the threshold can be increased to 70 or even 80 percent. Nonthreshold expenditures, on the other hand, can be reviewed on a decentralized basis, for example, within a single organization or department.

A formal one-batch review process facilitates direct comparison of competing capital initiatives using uniform criteria. Projects are reviewed and capital allocation is approved once a year. Conversely, when capital is meted out on an ongoing, serial basis, the approval process must invariably be done

> **SIDEBAR 4-1. Components of a Business Plan**
>
> - A project description, specifying facilities, equipment, services, location, and dollars.
> - A description of how the proposed initiative fits within the organization's current strategic development philosophy and mission.
> - A market assessment sufficient to provide a good sense of the dynamics of the market and its competitors as well as a rationale for volume, service, and revenue projections.
> - An implementation plan that delineates key tasks, dates, and challenges of implementation.
> - A five-year financial analysis. This includes an income statement, balance sheets, and statements of changes in financial position. Sufficient detail should be supplied for the reader to understand the assumptions underlying the numbers, and the process should highlight the variables critical to the project's success.
> - An assessment of project risk and related quantification of those risks.
> - A strategy for modification and termination. This should identify appropriate warning signals and delineate the steps that would be taken to limit the organization's risk.
>
> Source: Kaufman, Hall & Associates, Inc. Used with permission.

piecemeal as well. This often results in approval of projects that compete strategically or that, in combination, introduce unacceptable financial risk. In contrast, a one-batch review process eases process management and provides complete control of the amount and type of capital expenditures. This results in an enhanced ability to ensure alignment between proposed capital investments and strategic goals.

Although batch (nonserial) evaluation of capital requests is key to an effective capital allocation process, the process structure must incorporate enough flexibility to accommodate the evaluation of occasional emergency and out-of-cycle requests. However, such off-cycle requests must be reviewed within the same rigorous, corporate finance–based context as those requests evaluated in the batch process.

Quantitative analysis using corporate finance–based techniques

Effective capital allocation depends on the competent use of quantitative techniques used in corporate finance. These include the consideration of risk, through techniques such as Monte Carlo simulation described in Concept Three, calculation of net cash available for capital, incremental cash flow projections, and discounted cash flow or net present value, based on the organization's weighted average cost of capital. The mechanics of selected techniques are described later in the chapter. Although capital allocation does involve some qualitative analysis, the use of rigorous quantitative techniques ensures a common language and outcomes or end points that can be compared for each project under consideration. Qualitative issues can be quantified by building risk assessment into the process. When push comes to shove, an organization's long-term viability and value comes from its ability to generate a financial return. Each project's return needs to be quantified. A positive return gives the organization the ability to invest in the next strategy. A consensus-driven approach to capital allocation—one focused on what may "feel good" and "look nice"—does not provide the quantitative measures necessary to evaluate financial return. Analytical techniques derived from the principles of corporate finance provide such measures.

Data-driven and team-based decision making

Quantitative analysis using corporate finance techniques provides the fact base for informed decision making about capital investment opportunities. With involvement of key stakeholders, organizations should establish criteria for the evaluation and selection of such opportunities and involve key team members in the process of ranking and scoring capital requests.

Most organizations include financial return as one of the significant decision-making criteria, but it is seldom relied on as the only criterion. Its weighting as a criterion varies by organization. Organizations clearly cannot carry a series of investment decisions that don't add value to the organization. Best practice capital allocation allows management discretion but uses quantitative, rigorous analytics to provide a financial context for all decisions.

Coordinated calendar and planning cycles

Effective allocation of capital requires the coordination of the organization's financial planning, budgeting, and allocation processes. The timing and structure for these processes should reflect their interdependent nature and must be rigorously observed for optimal effectiveness. Rigorous calendar management is vital to ensure that projects or initiatives do not slip in and out of the process without comprehensive strategic and financial review. The comprehensive calendar should be communicated on an ongoing basis, and all staff should be aware of when capital requests and related analyses are due and are being evaluated.

Figure 4-1 illustrates the integration of the strategic planning, budgeting, capital allocation, and approval processes. From strategic plan development to ultimate capital approval, this decision-making cycle takes a full year to complete. Typically, strategic planning takes three to five months, followed by quantification and integration of identified initiatives in the financial planning process over the next two months. This leaves approximately five to seven months to complete the budgeting and capital allocation processes.

At the completion of the best practice cycle, management is able to present for board approval a coordinated and completely coherent presentation of the following:

- the five-year strategic plan,
- the long-term financial plan based on the strategic plan, and
- an operating and current-year capital budget based on the first year of the multiyear plans and incorporating the broader capital allocation decisions.

Keeping these interrelated decision-making processes tied to a firm calendar ensures consistent and comprehensive evaluation by management throughout the year. As Figure 4-1 reveals, capital allocation is an integral part of the organization's decision-making cycle.

A best practice approach to capital allocation takes into consideration the organization's decision-making style and culture. It must be flexible enough to be adapted as necessary and allow for a multiyear implementation

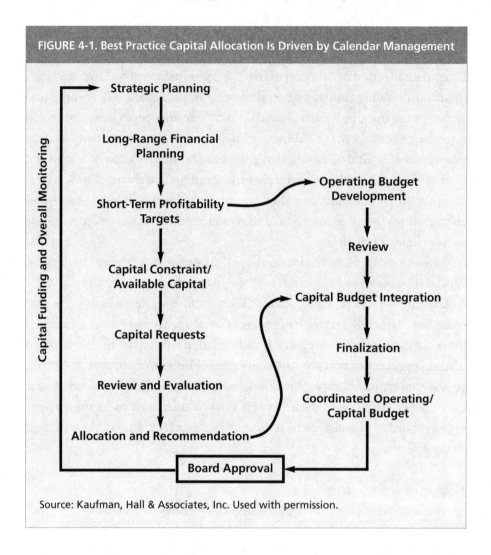

FIGURE 4-1. Best Practice Capital Allocation Is Driven by Calendar Management

Source: Kaufman, Hall & Associates, Inc. Used with permission.

time frame. Most healthcare organizations do not try to tackle the full process during the first year. Implementation over two to three years helps create buy-in and institutionalization of the approach as part of the organization's decision-making process.

Clear definition of available capital

How much can the organization afford to spend on capital investments? Every organization faces a limitation on its capital resources. Such a limitation is determined by the organization's current operations, debt structure, and cash position. To make informed and timely decisions, this limit—the capital constraint—must be well understood. Some organizations simply look at the income statement (for example, net income plus depreciation or a percentage of total operating revenue) as a starting point. This incomplete picture of capital availability can lead to financially detrimental levels of capital expenditures. To be complete, all sources and uses of funds, including principal payments, working capital changes, and additions to balance sheet cash reserves, must be added to the income statement–based calculation. If this complete calculation is used, the remaining sum is the net cash available for capital, or the capital constraint.

To define the capital constraint, start by asking the following simple question: "What amount of capital are we reasonably sure we can provide to support the organization's development over a defined period of time?" This relates to how much the organization can and should borrow as well as the level of cash that it can generate and retain from operations in uncertain times. The next step is to confirm specific targets for cash, debt service coverage, and debt-to-capitalization ratios established in the financial plan and then to translate these into annual goals. Next, the organization's debt capacity can be reconfirmed based on current-year operations and a five-year financial projection scenario to which the organization can commit. A table itemizing sources and uses of capital provides a complete picture of capital availability.

High level of governance, education, and communication

Governance is the linchpin to success of a capital allocation process. Having the operational executive team participate in a peer-review structure as an explicit component of project approval is critical to success. Peers know the questions to ask and will not accept incomplete responses or platitudes. They can help make the scarcity of resources real for colleagues.

The successful rollout of a high-quality capital allocation process requires commitment to that process throughout the organization. As mentioned earlier, commitment must originate from the top leaders and pervade all levels of management. Ensuring that organizational constituencies have a strong knowledge base about the principles of corporate finance and understand the capital allocation process also helps build commitment.

The entire management team must have at least a basic understanding of the corporate finance concepts embodied in effective decision making. All too often, capital allocation is viewed as strictly a finance function. However, experience shows that including nonfinancial managers is critical to effective, best practice capital allocation. Although analytical tools used in corporate finance may be new to some and may require education and training, particularly for department manager–level staff, it is absolutely critical to ensure that such education is provided on an ongoing basis. Increased knowledge about tools and techniques directed beyond the finance department and into line-management positions will help ensure institutionalization of the best practice capital allocation process.

Comprehensive communication of all aspects of the process—including steps in the allocation process, process methodologies, basic principles of corporate finance, project-based analysis, and the process calendar—is essential to success. Communication routes must be both broad and deep, including the board of directors, senior management, department directors, and clinicians. Up-front communication should provide a full description of the structure of the allocation process, including its objectives, timing, informational requirements, and approval structure. As the allocation process unfolds, a continuous stream of ongoing communication should be disseminated to all levels of the organization. This ensures proper usage of support tools, timely project analysis, consistency of technical approach, and correction of process or technical errors in an expeditious manner. As difficulties in the process are identified, communication provides the feedback essential for updating and correcting the allocation process used organizationwide.

Effective supporting materials are vital as an ongoing reference. Written materials describing the process and how to participate offer an effective implementation tool and can also provide basic information on corporate finance principles. The target of such materials should be middle management and senior management. Including clinical staff in the education process can empower clinicians to generate ideas, perform financial analysis, and present their projects within the structure of the allocation process. This minimizes end runs around the process.

Decentralizing the allocation process will increase its efficiency and effectiveness. To accomplish broad decentralization, the use of organizational

SIDEBAR 4-2. Barriers to Successful Rollout and Strategies to Overcome Such Barriers

- *Avoidance*: Expressed as "The process involves too much work," this barrier can be overcome by indicating that the project under consideration represents a significant investment. If the project is not worth the up-front analysis, why is it worth the investment?
- *Misperception*: Expressed as "My project is different," this barrier can be overcome through use of the common language of net present value (NPV). Not all projects will have a positive NPV, but through the objective quantification of financial return, each will be evaluated on an equal footing.
- *Misunderstanding*: Expressed as "This is a defensive project—its benefits cannot be quantified," this barrier can be overcome by indicating that all projects can be quantified and by quantifying the cost of not investing in the project. Organizations can use a portfolio approach, evaluating whether the portfolio as a whole adds value to the organization.
- *Subversion*: Expressed as "I will just go to the CEO—the CEO always approves what I want," this barrier can be overcome by the CEO's use of the formal capital allocation process as a means to say "no." The process forces decisions out of the hallway or private office and into the conference room.

Source: Kaufman, Hall & Associates, Inc. Used with permission.

champions to support implementation and provide an ongoing resource can be very successful.

Typical barriers to successful rollout and strategies to overcome such barriers are shown in Sidebar 4-2.

Process integrity through project monitoring and measurement

Ongoing measurement of actual investment performance must be built into process governance as well. Such measurement provides credibility, enabling specific comparison of actual results to projected results. In addition, because individuals know they will be held accountable for performance results, the quality of up-front analysis is greatly improved and more realistic. Ongoing measurement also provides a means for transferring knowledge about investment success or failure throughout the organization.

Once an organization establishes a capital budget, staff should review performance from operations each and every quarter, comparing performance to the budget from a cash flow perspective. Is net income plus depreciation less principal payments and working capital tracking to budget? If so, the organization may increase balance sheet cash reserves or increase allocated capital to support other projects that did not make the initial allocation. If cash flow performance is worse than budgeted, the organization will need to scale back its capital spending.

Post-project monitoring helps ensure that cost and revenue projections are on target and are reasonable. Organizations must compare actual outcomes of approved investments with budgeted results. This ensures the integrity of the analytic and decision-making process. Project analysis should always include an exit strategy with a defined point at which the plug is pulled on investments that are not performing up to defined expectations.

Implementation of a smoothly running best practice capital allocation process is likely to be a two- or three-year process. During the first year, managers buy into the process as a step in the right direction. During the second year, they learn to live within the process and learn how to apply it to all areas. By year three, the best practice capital allocation process is just a part of what managers do. They now automatically screen bad projects from the process and understand the critical link between strategic and financial planning.

To evaluate implementation progress, leaders should ask the following questions: Has the number of projects coming in through the "back door" been reduced or eliminated? Have departments or disciplines that have always proposed highly suspect, but politically palatable, projects become less visible since the rigorous capital allocation process was implemented? Has the quality of project analysis improved since standardized project-review requirements were established? Has the general caliber of the submitted projects improved? Are the projects focused more on market growth and overall return?

If the answer to any or all of these questions is yes, the organization has made significant progress toward successful implementation of corporate finance–based capital allocation. The ultimate goal of a best practice capital allocation process is to deploy the organization's capital in a way that is

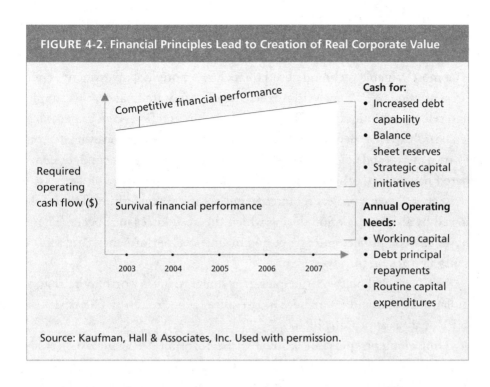

FIGURE 4-2. Financial Principles Lead to Creation of Real Corporate Value

Source: Kaufman, Hall & Associates, Inc. Used with permission.

most likely to support the organization's overall strategy and generate additional capital for future investment. Performance at a survival-only level may not actually ensure future survival, and it certainly does not achieve competitive performance (see Figure 4-2). Every small step taken toward that ultimate goal helps the organization improve its competitive financial position and enables it to pursue aggressive and effective strategies.

The capital allocation process must be designed to evolve and change over time. The process should be reviewed annually to assess its progress toward meeting specified goals. This involves looking at what works and why, what does not work and why, what needs to be added, and what components are unnecessary and can be eliminated. Review of the process, in fact, should be a formal component of the process structure and should occur at approximately the same time each year. Organizations should be willing and able to adjust the process to meet that organization's needs. For example, adjustments may need to be made to the schedule, analytical components, and dollar thresholds. Individuals participating in the process at both the leadership and department levels should be empowered to make necessary changes to enhance the process.

Net Present Value Analysis

The most valuable technique used to analyze a potential investment is net present value (NPV) analysis. At the core of corporate finance, this simple and reliable technique distills the financial ebbs and flows of a project to a single dollar value. Because it does so, it enables a project to be evaluated on its own merits and helps answer the question of how the project might compare financially to others under consideration.

Generally, each project requires an initial capital expenditure. This is followed by a start-up period during which financial losses may occur. Then, hopefully, the project enters a period of financial performance that represents a return on the investment.

NPV is based on two principles: (1) a dollar today is worth more than a dollar next year and (2) higher risks require higher rewards. The basics of NPV analysis appear in Sidebar 4-3.

Four elements must be known to perform an NPV analysis: (1) an estimate of the up-front investment, (2) projection of free cash flows, (3) a cost of capital estimate, and (4) a terminal value estimate. Each is described below.

Estimate of the up-front investment

An estimate of the up-front investment should be reasonably clear if a proper business plan has been developed for the project. Be sure to look only at incremental expenditures, ignoring outlays already made. These, in effect, are sunk costs—costs already incurred. Do not neglect to include opportunity costs, which are proceeds lost by foregoing other opportunities. For example, if the project is a building that is to be constructed on land that could be sold for a certain price, the value of the land should be considered. Consider also working capital requirements, such as operating expenses, that will need to be paid from cash reserves before the project is able to carry these expenses on its own.

SIDEBAR 4-3. Calculating Net Present Value

The future value of a present sum of money is expressed as $FV = PV (1+r)^t$ where:

> FV = Future value
>
> PV = Present value
>
> r = Interest rate
>
> t = Number of time periods

By rearranging the above terms, it is possible to express the present value of a future cash flow as follows:

$$PV = \frac{FV}{(1 + r)^t}$$

The present value of an investment decision that results in a series of future cash flows may be expressed as follows:

$$NPV = C_0 + \frac{C_1}{(1 + r)^t} + \frac{C_2}{(1 + r)^2} + \frac{C_n}{(1 + r)^n}$$

where

> NPV = Net present value
>
> C_0 = Up-front expenditure associated with the investment
>
> $C_0, C_2 \dots C_n$ = Particular cash flows expected in particular periods
>
> r = Interest (or discount) rate

As an example, assume that an invesment of $50 now would yield cash flows of $25 per year for three years and that the discount rate is 10 percent. The NPV of that investment would be:

$$(\$50) + \frac{\$25}{1.1} + \frac{\$25}{(1.1)^2} + \frac{\$25}{(1.1)^3} = (\$50) + \$23 + \$21 + \$19 = \$13$$

In corporate finance theory, the decision rule is that the investment is acceptable if it has a positive NPV, because this means that the investment generates more than the opportunity cost of capital.

Projection of free cash flows

A projection of free cash flows involves determining how much cash is generated in a particular year—cash that could be available to distribute to an investor. Free cash flow is equal to net income plus depreciation minus increases in working capital requirements minus capital expenditures. Depreciation and allocation of existing corporate overhead should not be considered in the projection. Because the cost of capital will be considered separately (see below), projections of free cash flows should also assume that the project is financed with equity. Therefore, interest or principal payments should not be included in the projections. Remember to explicitly estimate the effect of incidental factors such as increased market share, incorporate the effects of inflation on revenues and expenses, and include ongoing capital requirements necessary to keep the project going.

Cost of capital estimate

The cost of capital involves determining the rate at which the cash flows should be discounted. If the project is risky, it should have a higher expected return than money invested in relatively risk-free investments. How should the discount rate be set to account for the risk of a particular investment? A wide diversity of answers to this question exists in both the business and healthcare communities. A number of methods can be used, but common to all methods is the conclusion that the real cost of capital is significantly higher than the cost of debt. Generally, the weighted average cost of capital is well recognized by investment bankers and financial consultants as an excellent proxy for the cost of capital for not-for-profit organizations. See Sidebar 4-4 for a demonstration of how to calculate the weighted average cost of capital.

Terminal value estimate

The terminal value of a project is the estimate of that investment's value after the original projection period. Terminal value often can account for 30 to 60 percent of the investment's total value. The calculation of terminal value can be approached in four ways:

SIDEBAR 4-4. Calculating the Weighted Average Cost of Capital

The weighted average cost of capital (WACC) can be expressed as

WACC = [R(e) x E] + [R(d) x D], where:

> R(e) = Cost of equity capital (see below)
> E = Percentage of equity in capital structure
> R(d) = Cost of debt
> D = Percentage of debt in capital structure

Cost of equity capital R(e) can be calculated as

> R(e) = R(f) + B[R(m) − R(f)], where

> R(f) = Risk-free rate (based, for example, on 30-year
> treasury yields)
> R(m) − R(f) = Marketwide risk premium
> B = Beta (risk)

For an example health system, the variables are as follows:

> R(e) = 16.05%
> E = 74.00%
> R(d) = 5.00%
> D = 26.00%
> R(f) = 6.449%
> R(m) − R(f) = 8.000%
> B = 1.20

Long-term debt is $1.3 billion; net assets are $3.7 billion.

The cost of equity capital equation, R(e) = R(f) + B[R(m) − R(f)], would read:
    16.05% = 6.449% + 1.20[8.000%].
The weighted average cost of capital equation, WACC = [R(e) x E] + [R(d) x D],
    would read: 13.18% = [16.05% x 74.00%] + [5.00% x 26.00%).
Note that as the beta or risk factor used in the equation increases, so does the
weighted average cost of capital. Therefore, with a beta of 1.30, for example,
the WACC is 13.77 percent. A beta of 1.50 yields a WACC of 14.95 percent.

1. Assume *no value*, which would be appropriate for an item such as a computer that has no material value at the end of the project life.
2. Calculate *liquidation value*, based on the assumption that the asset has an anticipated sale value at the end of the project life.
3. Calculate *annuity/perpetuity value*, which assumes that the investment will continue to generate free cash flow equal to that of the last year of the projection period during a period ranging from one year to forever.
4. Calculate *growth perpetuity value*, which is similar to the perpetuity value but includes an assumption that the level of free cash flow after the projection period will change.

Remember that the terminal value of the project accrues at the end of the projection period, so to define its present value, it must be discounted at the same discount rate back to the beginning of the projection period.

Project Selection

According to corporate finance theory, the traditional way to select projects is to rank them, placing the project with the highest NPV first. This is followed by projects of lesser NPV in order of value. According to this approach, all projects with a positive NPV are selected, and those with a negative NPV are discarded.

Some organizations establish a weighting system that captures mission, strategy, and financial issues in a composite ranking. Independent of the weighting system used, however, all truly effective ranking procedures list the projects in a complete table in descending order of NPV. Such a table allows an organization to consider the list as a whole. Does the list have a positive or negative NPV? If the organization selects this list of projects, however that decision is made, is the organization adding to or detracting from its value?

As your understanding of the essential concepts of corporate finance increases, you can begin to combine principles to further focus and sharpen the analysis. For example, ranking projects by NPV has been a staple of corporate-style capital allocation since the 1950s. However, NPV analysis can be made more powerful by integrating the Monte Carlo simulation techniques described in Concept Three. Using simulation to further analyze projects creates a much more accurate estimate of risk-adjusted value, which statisticians call *expected net present value* (ENPV).

For example, your hospital is thinking of developing a second cardiac catheterization lab. After following the analytic methods suggested in this chapter, the NPV of the project is estimated to be $750,000 based on the expected demand and assumed operating costs. Using simulation techniques, you can estimate a range of possible NPVs based on hundreds or thousands of scenarios involving uncertain demand and other assumptions with unpredictable outcomes. Although the NPV associated with the original point estimates was $750,000, this is not necessarily the average or expected NPV. Simulation will provide a range of NPV outcomes of all combinations of demand and operating assumptions to create the ENPV. The ENPV provides an indication of the investment's likely return, incorporating risk, and illuminates potential hidden risks even in projects with high ENPV. Ranking the portfolio of projects by simulated ENPV may give you an entirely different and more accurate view of the selection decision than that provided by point estimates.

The proper evaluation of projects and their selection for your portfolio may not be an easy process financially or politically. Applying principles of corporate finance, however, immeasurably enhances the decision-making process. A well-developed and implemented capital allocation process using these principles ensures your organization's future ability to play ball and live its mission.

Case Example: Capital Allocation in Practice

This example describes one organization's recent implementation of a corporate finance–based capital allocation process. Although the name of the organization is fictitious, the information provided is real.

The organization at a glance

Alpha Health System (AHS) is the largest healthcare network in the state. A fully integrated system covering the north and central regions of the state, AHS owns and operates 11 acute care hospitals. The system has 2,000 licensed beds and a staff of nearly 9,600 employees. The system's non–acute care operations include skilled nursing facilities, senior housing facilities, home care agencies, occupational health services, hospices, primary care clinics, fitness facilities, and a 150,000-member preferred provider organization. AHS generates approximately $1.7 billion in annual gross revenue and is rated "A2" by Moody's Investors Service.

Previous capital allocation process

The capital allocation process in place at AHS during the late 1990s and early 2000s resembled the process used by many healthcare organizations. The amount of capital available to support the organization's development during a specified time period—the capital constraint—was devised by looking at the annual cash budget rather than by considering the organization's total capital capacity and long-range financial plan.

Financial planning had a firm place in AHS's culture (the good news), but it was not as rigorous as that offered by a corporate finance–based approach (the bad news). The process used to evaluate and approve proposed capital investments was as follows. Each facility or entity in the system prepared a three- to five-year plan, outlining major projects and capital needs. The corporate finance team used these lists to prepare a matrix of the wish lists by facility/entity, by item, and by year. The management executive committee reviewed the wish-list matrix and, having calculated the capital constraint and being aware of the dollars available to be spent, determined how much and where capital dollars would be spent.

In the AHS process, routine and strategic capital items were segregated. The system allocated routine capital based on historical spending patterns. Strategic capital was defined as "all projects in excess of $500,000." These were often lump sums of unidentified, loosely defined individual projects (for example, "new facilities for $2.0 million"). As a result of this allocation approach, routine capital requests drove the dollars available for allocation to strategic capital requirements.

Financial analysis of projects was limited. Detailed analyses generally were not prepared until immediately before beginning a project or expending the funds and thus were not critical to the up-front project evaluation. Projects were approved in a serial fashion, which meant that project funding could disappear if the organization's financial performance changed before a project started drawing on funds. Without the consistent and simultaneous comparative evaluation of multiple projects, it was very difficult for AHS to optimize its portfolio of capital investment opportunities. In addition, without a formal process for making capital allocation decisions, the management executive committee often made decisions based solely on subjective and, at times, unstated criteria.

The impetus for a new process

A number of factors provided the impetus for a new capital allocation process. Like all healthcare organizations in the late 1990s and early 2000s, AHS was concerned about lack of net revenue growth. Managed care reimbursement constraints and the effects of the Balanced Budget Act had created considerable pressure on net revenue. Quite simply, fewer dollars were coming into the system. Yet routine and strategic capital requests continued at a high level and were growing, creating a disparity between the dollars available to meet capital needs and those requested. Because operations were not able to generate additional return, the system relied increasingly on investment returns from selected capital projects to maintain profitability and liquidity targets.

When income from operations and investment returns began to slide, AHS leaders started to express concern about the serial approach to project approval. They recognized that the projects on the radar screen first, in fact, may not be those of the highest strategic priority or with the highest potential return for the organization. Had they evaluated the whole group of projects on the front end, the leaders acknowledged that the mix of projects receiving funding might have been quite different. In late 2002, AHS leaders embraced the need to create a rigorous capital allocation process based on corporate finance principles.

Redesign objectives

The key objectives for redesigning the existing capital allocation process were to provide for

- objective decision making;
- a fixed, predetermined process;
- enhanced and decentralized analysis;
- comparative review of projects; and
- quantification of decision making.

To address these objectives, AHS established a task force of key financial and operating leaders. This approach helped to ensure organization-wide participation in process design, sensitivity to operating and management issues generated by various design options, and ownership of the new process. Task force members included the executive vice president of hospital operations, the senior vice president of regional hospital operations, the system's CFO, two major hospital CEOs (one from an urban hospital and one from a regional hospital), the senior vice president (VP) of ambulatory services, the medical director, and three members of the corporate finance staff.

Process redesign

The task force concentrated its capital allocation process redesign efforts in five distinct areas. The first was to *define the principles and objectives of a systemwide approach to capital allocation*. The group identified the need to disconnect current capital allocation from past spending patterns. The historical benchmark approach did not allow the organization to respond adequately to changing market and financial conditions. Further, a status quo approach impeded consideration of potentially promising new investment opportunities. The task force also focused on the need for equal access to system-generated dollars for capital projects. Each entity in the system would have access to the system's total available dollars through a well-defined and well-articulated capital allocation process for the system as a whole.

Next, the task force *redefined how to calculate the capital constraint*, agreeing that a specific calculation would cover all capital requirements, not simply available cash. The team's capital constraint calculation appears as Figure 4-3. Note that the "Uses of Cash" portion includes a systemwide 10 percent capital-contingency pool for emergencies. The task force also segregated cash uses into those below (nonthreshold) or above a minimum dollar threshold (threshold capital). For ease of implementation, AHS retained $500,000 as its evaluation threshold and agreed to reevaluate that dollar sum on an annual basis. A complete financial analysis was required for all projects with a cost of $500,000 or greater. Approximately $14 million of the cash available for capital was allocated to fund nonthreshold capital requests and a significantly larger $23 million to threshold capital requests. This split was expected to help ensure that routine and small requests did not make up too large a piece of the total capital pie.

The third task tackled by the team was to *create a means to allocate dollars for nonthreshold capital to system entities* in a way that would reward performance. This would remove the subjectivity of a political approach to capital allocation and provide financial support to meet minimum needs. Departmentally generated capital requests would continue to be managed locally, but the dollars available to the entity for such capital would now be allocated based on the long-term profitability of the requesting entity as measured by EBIDA. Nonprofitable, non–revenue generating, and small entities would receive a minimum allocation of the available nonthreshold capital to fund vital needs. All entities were provided data on the design of nonthreshold capital allocation so that no "gaming" would occur. Figure 4-4 provides a look at this allocation.

The task force's fourth area of focus was to *establish consistent analytical standards for all threshold projects*. The task force communicated the analytic requirements systemwide and encouraged decentralized analysis. The system's investment in state-of-the-art financial decision software and educational efforts supporting the software and its tools made decentralized analysis possible and, indeed, expected within each entity.

The task force's final task was to *create a practical schedule*. To this end, the task force defined a process calendar that was consistent and integrated with the organization's ongoing planning and implementation processes. AHS committed to a calendar-driven approach to planning and implementation (as represented in Figure 4-1), codified that approach, and communicated specific timing requirements systemwide. During 2003, the first year of implementation, the calendar was modified somewhat to provide extra time for proper project analysis.

FIGURE 4-3. The Capital Constraint Calculation	
Sources of cash	**2002 Strategic Financial Plan ($000s)**
Operating income	17,249
Add: Depreciation and amortization	49,381
Other income sources (uses)	(2,975)
Use of funded depreciation	10,000
Total sources of cash	**73,655**
Uses of cash	
Retirement of long-term debt	(11,737)
Increase in working capital	(18,554)
Carryover from prior year approvals of capital	(3,130)
Total uses of cash (excluding capital)	**(33,421)**
Total cash available for capital	**40,234**
Less 10% emergency capital contingency	(4,023)
Net cash available for allocation	**36,211**
Less cash allocated to nonthreshold capital	(13,608)
Cash available for threshold capital	**$22,602**

Source: Kaufman, Hall & Associates, Inc. Used with permission.

A capital allocation council was chartered as the system's decision-making body. The council included AHS's CEO, chief operating officer, CFO, senior VP of operations, and a physician VP of one of the facilities. "The goal was to avoid a large-group capital allocation decision-making process that would involve various constituencies with different agendas and different axes to grind," describes AHS's VP of finance who served the council in a support role.

FIGURE 4-4. Allocation of Nonthreshold Capital

Department	Adjusted EBITDA	Allocable EBITDA	% of Total EBITDA	Allocation of $13,608	Allocation Adjustments to Minimum ($)	Allocation of $13,608	Final Allocation Percentage
Hospital A	$38,373	$38,373	38.3	$5,206	—	$4,394	32.3
Hospital B	29,839	29,839	29.8	4,049	—	3,417	25.1
Hospital C	13,530	13,530	13.5	1,836	—	1,549	11.4
Hospital D	5,060	5,060	5.0	687	—	579	4.3
Hospital E	340	340	0.3	46	$125	125	0.9
Hospital F	905	905	0.9	123	125	125	0.9
Hospital G	3,118	3,118	3.1	423	750	750	5.5
Hospital H	845	845	0.8	115	370	370	2.7
Hospital I	—	—	0.0	—	—	—	0.0
Hospital J	8,286	8,286	8.3	1,124	—	949	7.0
Hospital K	—	—	0.0	—	—	—	0.0
Central business office	—	—	0.0	—	100	100	0.7
Laundry	—	—	0.0	—	100	100	0.7
Information systems	—	—	0.0	—	750	750	5.5
Corporate services	(45,549)	—	0.0	—	400	400	2.9
Education	—	—	0.0	—	—	—	0.0
Alpha Health centers	—	—	0.0	—	—	—	0.0
Total AHS	**$54,747**	**$100,296**	**100.0%**	**$13,608**	**$2,720**	**$13,608**	**100.0**

Source: Kaufman, Hall & Associates, Inc. Used with permission.

Meeting implementation challenges and evaluating the new process

2003: Year one

During its first year, AHS's new corporate finance–based capital allocation process achieved two major accomplishments: (1) improved analysis and (2) enhanced support of the decision-making process. Project champions in entities throughout the system were able to prepare appropriate and improved analyses. "To devise realistic reimbursement assumptions, for example, the reimbursement staff needed to understand a proposed project and carefully think through how the project would be reimbursed. Global assumptions may not have been applicable," notes the system's VP of finance. Decentralized analyses ensured accurate and detailed financial input.

Training time related to the analytics was required during the first year for both corporate and facility-based staff. "Everyone needed to understand that politics were being removed from the capital allocation process. To some extent, it took failure to get a project approved in year one for staff to understand the magnitude of the change," recalls the VP of finance.

With individual and comparative project data at its fingertips, the capital allocation council was able to make better-informed decisions. Using the software's decision support structure, the council used qualitative and quantitative criteria to develop a capital investment portfolio. The review criteria were weighted: two-thirds weight was assigned to financial criteria; one-third was related to other criteria such as community service and physician issues. "This weighting made approval of an unprofitable project an explicit event, visible to everyone in the system," says the VP of finance.

As it continually revised the structure of the selected portfolio, the software enabled the council to see the quantitative impact of its decisions on a real-time basis. The VP of finance explains: "Use of a best practice capital allocation process enabled us to look at the whole picture. If the analytics for a certain project showed that the project would not meet financial criteria, but the capital allocation council felt the project needed to be approved for community service reasons, we now knew what the financial shortfall would be and could address how to balance or make up for that shortfall." Everyone became aware of the financial consequences of the decisions they were making.

Fewer projects made it to the table for discussion. Instead of extensive wish lists, only projects that were able to pass the rigor of the local review process were submitted for consideration. "In the first year alone, perhaps 15 projects never made it to the capital allocation council because the staff didn't want to go through the analytics or thought that the project could not 'survive' the analysis," says the VP of finance. A project evaluation form, an important tool included in the state-of-the art software, added discipline to the analyses. Because everyone used the same method of presenting and evaluating a project, a direct apples-to-apples comparison was possible.

The efficiency of the new process encouraged members of the capital allocation council and system managers alike. In an all-day meeting scheduled to review 58 projects, the capital allocation council not only covered its agenda, but finished earlier than expected. The review process was not an agonizing, exhausting one because the information needed for decision making was in front of everyone. Managers throughout the system thought the process was fair, and even if an entity's project was not approved, its champions understood why. After the first year of implementation, AHS leaders were satisfied that corporate finance–based capital allocation represented a step in the right direction.

2004: Year two

During the second year of implementation, AHS focused on fine-tuning the new capital allocation process, concentrating on such areas as the criteria used to allocate capital to the corporate office and the structure of access to contingency funds. The AHS corporate office includes capital-intensive areas, such as the financial operations, information technology, centralized billing, and a laundry. Because these operations do not produce cash flow, the task force needed to find a means other than EBIDA to make appropriate amounts of capital available to them.

During the first year of the new process, AHS wrestled with how to handle capital allocated to the corporate office. "In year one, we set a lower level of $25,000 for corporate's threshold capital. This was a mistake because so many more projects now needed to be reviewed," says the VP of finance. During year two, AHS reconfigured the nonthreshold allocation by fixing a minimum allocation to the corporate office and each component operation and applying the consistent $500,000 threshold to corporate projects. In effect, services such as information technology and the corporate billing office became their own entities subject to the same threshold capital requirements of all other facilities.

In the area of the emergency capital contingency, AHS increased the size of the contingency to ensure control of total capital spending and empha-sized substitution of capital projects as a first means to meet emergency or out-of-cycle needs. The capital allocation council strictly controlled access to contingency funds.

Year two benefits included the following:

- even better project analysis by champions and champion teams,
- continued self-imposed weeding out of marginal projects by the individual entities before reaching the capital allocation council,
- reduced corporate project review requirements, and
- increased focus by senior management to maintain the integrity of the process.

After the second year of implementation, AHS leaders were satisfied that they had fully applied the fundamentals of the corporate finance–based capital allocation process and had learned how to apply it to nongrowth areas, such as corporate office functions. "We now knew how many dollars we could spend and could make capital allocation deci-sions based on solid financial criteria. The quantitative analysis provided a real comfort level about the bottom line results we could achieve," says the VP of finance.

Areas for continued vigilance and future efforts

By year three (2005), corporate finance–based capital allocation has become "just a part of what we do" at AHS. However, continued vigilance is required in the future. Leaders must stick to the decisions made during the allocation process. To facilitate this, decision makers are informed on a month-to-month basis about how each decision affects AHS's long-term financial success.

AHS leaders also recognize the need to follow through to monitor the projects selected for funding. Actual project progress must be tracked against project analyses submitted at the approval stage. Data related to project-specific performance must be captured and analyzed. Project updates must be required as a part of the capital requests submitted in subsequent years. The financial impact of decisions made and potential changes to those decisions must be quantified on an ongoing basis. "Information related to assumptions that did or did not turn out to be true needs to be available and reviewed before the next capital allocation process begins," says the VP of finance.

Future efforts at AHS will focus on the following:

- continuing education to broaden and deepen analytical capabilities systemwide,
- increasing sophistication of project monitoring,
- using portfolio management techniques to ensure the best possible mix of capital projects, and
- extending the process to the individual unit level for application to nonthreshold capital projects.

In year three of the new capital allocation process, AHS leaders are firmly committed to the belief that guessing just does not work anymore. A rigorous, corporate finance–based capital allocation process is the only way to effectively integrate long-term strategies and current-year capital investment.

A special note of thanks to the AHS's VP of finance who helped tell this story in a way that would be helpful to other healthcare organizations.

CONCEPT FIVE

Strategic Budgeting

Jason H. Sussman

THE BUDGETING PROCESS. Often the bane of existence for healthcare financial managers, it can be a time-consuming and unfulfilling process involving confrontation, negotiation, and politics. For some organizations, budgeting fully consumes half of the fiscal year. The effect? The organization's financial management team and tools are essentially unavailable to support key strategic needs. In addition, the final budget is often not in line with the organization's strategic financial interests.

Such misapplication of organizational resources cannot be tolerated in the current healthcare environment. Decision making in healthcare organizations must be fully supported by a top-notch financial team, comprehensive financial analysis, and a well-integrated strategic financial plan.

Overview of Strategic Budgeting

Strategic budgeting is a best practice approach characterized by the integration of strategic and financial planning, capital planning, and a "connected" budget development process. Founded on principles of corporate finance as described throughout this book, strategic budgeting is critical to integrated decision making. Its foundation lies in the explicit quantification of the organization's strategies in operating and capital plans framed by specific, measurable targets and objectives. A best practice budget translates strategies directly to operating targets. Both nonfinancial and financial managers then monitor and measure performance against those targets. As a result, they are well equipped to proactively identify trends that require attention to ensure the organization's ongoing success.

A common approach to healthcare budgeting, which is *not* the best practice, recommended approach, is a combination "top down/bottom up" process. Essentially, executives at the senior management level centrally establish all significant budget targets, but the actual budget is completed at the departmental level.

The *top down* portion of the process occurs when the leadership team sets annual profitability targets. For organizations not engaged in corporate finance–based strategic financial planning, this typically resembles more of an art than a science. In some organizations, this year's target is based on last year's performance. Others set their targets based on information gleaned from various industry periodicals. Still others use the profitability levels achieved by peer organizations and competitors as a guide to their own targets. In any case, without a financial planning foundation, the targets established by senior management are not necessarily consistent with the organization's strategic goals and related capital needs.

In an attempt to make the process efficient, budget directives are passed down to department managers. Because there is often limited communication, operations-level staff (the people who make the budget happen) are uninformed as to why targeted levels of operations are necessary vis-à-vis the organization's overall strategy. With limited understanding of the targets' strategic foundation, the overall budget does not gain the support of the operations-level staff.

Having established the overall budget targets, the *bottom up* portion of the process begins as staff embark on a multimonth exercise to develop the detailed annual budget. Department managers submit budget requests for the coming year based on budget directives provided by the executive team. Unfortunately, because such individuals may be disconnected from and uninformed about the organization's overall strategic and financial goals, the proposals developed often reflect individual departmental requirements. This invariably results in an initial budget that is way off the mark because of reasons described in Sidebar 5-1.

> **SIDEBAR 5-1. Possible Reasons for Inaccurate Budgets Using the Typical Budgeting Approach**
>
> - Proposed departmental budget purposefully *overestimates* expenses to ensure that the department retains sufficient budget dollars following the inevitable negotiations to pare initial budget requests.
> - Proposed departmental budget *underestimates* expenses because of lack of awareness of new strategic directions or expansion plans that will affect their portions of the operation.
> - Proposed departmental budget *low balls* expenses so that new strategic initiatives emerging during the year must be funded by other parts of the organization.
> - Proposed departmental budget presents a *pie in the sky* wish list.
>
> Source: Kaufman, Hall & Associates, Inc. Used with permission.

Thus, the next step in the approach—the paring or cutting and negotiation process—begins. Financial managers try to determine what each department really needs to operate. A clarification process ensues, complete with frequent, confusing, sometimes acrimonious, and time-consuming meetings. Participants slog through this stage, which often gets so convoluted that many lose faith in the numbers that emerge. A huge amount of time is invested by all those with a stake in the budget.

Unlike the budget described earlier, the strategic budget is an integrated implementation plan that directly connects the organization's mission and strategic objectives to the day-to-day efforts of its staff. Such budgeting ensures management's active control and direction of the capital management cycle (see Figure 1-1 in Concept One).

As described in Concept One, the cycle includes three major, integrally connected planning functions: strategic, financial, and capital planning. Plans in each area, developed in the cycle's first phase, help executives focus on the best possible investment of the organization's resources. The multi-year strategic plan incorporates specific market initiatives for the coming year. The financial plan quantifies the potential capital and operating requirements of those strategies and establishes the annual financial targets required to fund the proposed strategies.

In the cycle's second phase, operating and capital budgets are developed and implemented, thereby "operationalizing" the planning framework. Based on the financial and strategic plans, these budgets outline specific recommendations for investing the capital needed to implement specific strategies and implementation costs in relation to income. Recommendations are consistent with targeted cash flow and short-term and long-term strategic financial plans.

The third and final phase of the cycle focuses on monitoring and tracking the goals established during the budgeting phase. If these goals are met, so are the organization's larger planning objectives. Relevant data related to operating performance is fed back to those performing the planning function as the cycle recommences for the next fiscal year.

Because the planning and budgeting processes are fully integrated, responsibility for developing and implementing the budget spans the entire organization. This enables the finance staff to apply its resources effectively and efficiently to support organizational decision making. Financial executives must ensure that the necessary processes are in place to enable managers to convert the organization's overall financial objectives into "on the ground" operating targets.

Eight Key Steps of Strategic Budgeting

The key steps of a best practice, integrated approach to budgeting are as follows:

Step 1: Develop the strategic and financial plans
Step 2: Communicate objectives
Step 3: Obtain/provide feedback about targets
Step 4: Develop a first-pass budget
Step 5: Review the first-pass budget
Step 6: Make adjustments and finalize the budget
Step 7: Use the budget as a management tool
Step 8: Restart the cycle

Each step is described in the next sections of this chapter.

Step 1: Develop the strategic and financial plans

During the first several months of the fiscal year, senior executives, often with the input of the board of directors, provide the impetus for the strategic budgeting process by defining or revising the organization's strategic and financial goals (Step 1). They identify strategic priorities and the financial targets to be achieved in pursuing these priorities. As described in Concept One, executives use the strategic plan to outline specific programs or services that should be pursued during the plan period. Through the strategic and financial planning process described in Concept Three, they assess the achievability of these initiatives. The financial plan includes capital, cash, and profitability targets. It also includes overall volume projections for the coming fiscal year—such as total patient days, discharges, changes in average length of stay, outpatient volume, and surgical volume—required to meet such targets.

Step 2: Communicate objectives

To gain buy-in, as the next step, executives communicate with department managers throughout the organization about strategic and financial goals, related operating imperatives, and how these were generated. This provides a common understanding of the organization's overall strategy and a clear foundation for operating or budgeting parameters, such as the need to hold staffing to current levels, increase surgical volume by A percent, increase salaries no more than B percent, reduce supply costs by C percent, or increase patient admissions by D percent. Without such a strategic foundation, staff often receive these parameters as little more than dictates. By providing department managers with the strategic context for concrete guidelines or targets, all managers can fully understand the consequences of meeting or not meeting the established targets.

Step 3: Obtain/provide feedback about targets

Next, executives give department managers the opportunity to provide feedback on the key assumptions underlying the strategic and financial targets.

During this step, managers have a real opportunity to validate the operational practicality of the goals described in the financial plan by answering questions such as the following:

- What activities are occurring in my department to help the organization achieve its strategic and financial objectives for the upcoming fiscal year?
- What is occurring or might occur in the department or among departments to prevent the organization from achieving its strategic and financial objectives for the upcoming fiscal year?

Sidebar 5-2 outlines the many benefits of this interactive dialog.

Department managers can often provide valuable input about how specific strategies are likely to affect their departments. For example, perhaps a healthcare system will be starting a new women's health service or a hospital will be buying a high-end piece of diagnostic equipment that is expected to increase outpatient volume by 3 percent. What are the departmental effects of such strategies? Knowledge about why certain targets are needed and how they support the success of the organization helps build buy-in at the operations level.

Step 4: Develop a first-pass budget

Incorporating feedback from Step 3, the senior team revises and translates volume projections into an overall financial and capital plan that delineates specific financial targets consistent with identified strategic imperatives. With a best practice approach to financial management, the specific targets of the financial plan drive initial budget development, in effect rolling the financial plan down through the organization.

During this next step, the finance team prepares a first-pass budget that translates the assumptions of the overall strategy into concrete statistical targets and departmental budgets. Data related to patient volume and other organizational drivers are derived from the strategic, financial, and capital plans. Core data used in financial planning—such as the projected number of outpatient visits, admissions, and discharges—are integrated within individual budgets and provided to department managers.

SIDEBAR 5-2. The Benefits of Dialog About Strategic and Financial Targets

- Enables executives to clarify any targets whose purpose may not be clear to managers
- Provides an opportunity for managers to help executives clearly define the interdepartmental impact of the defined initiatives
- Effectively breaks down the "silo" mentality that typically occurs during a budgeting process
- Expands ownership of the organization's strategic plan
- Creates real accountability for the plan's operational integration

Source: Kaufman, Hall & Associates, Inc. Used with permission.

For example, consider a hospital that is planning to build a new heart center. The organization's financial plan identifies expected incremental increases in inpatient and outpatient volumes associated with this initiative. The financial plan also quantifies incremental operating costs and capital expenses related to the purchase of diagnostic equipment and facility construction. But how does the hospital's finance team operationalize this initiative for the radiology department, for example?

The team obtains data that show the relationship between overall inpatient and outpatient activity levels and activity levels in radiology (for example, the number of exams per average admission or the number of x-rays per average patient day). These relationships could be derived from actual data or could be estimated based on the experience of others. Specific departmental costs can be identified as fixed or variable relative to volume. Applying these parameters, new cardiovascular admissions projected in the strategic financial plan can be correlated to a specific number of radiology exams. In turn, these new exams will drive quantifiable requirements for increases in staffing, supplies, utilities, and so forth in the radiology department.

Each department has a primary cost-per-unit statistic that is tied to assumptions included in the overall strategy. For example, the laboratory's core statistic is lab procedures as a percentage of patient days. Through use of software that integrates strategic assumptions with budget development, these relationships are held constant. When the leadership team indicates that patient days will go up or down, inpatient and outpatient lab procedures will also go up or down on the budget provided to the lab director.

Hence, this initial budget provides managers with line-item budget detail tied directly to the organization's overall financial strategy. Requirements related to new and ongoing strategic initiatives are specifically quantified.

Step 5: Review the first-pass budget

At this point, department managers are asked to review the first-pass budgets that include their department-specific targets. Because department managers now understand the link between achieving budget targets and the organization's overall strategic success, this review, which occurs within no more than a month-long time frame, is a critical one. The role of department managers is to identify necessary exceptions and to define specific, measurable alternatives that will offset such exceptions to keep the departmental and organizational budgets balanced. They review and adjust the first-pass budget in the context of the predefined overall targets reflecting required, integrated organizational and departmental performance. This process forces all managers to assume responsibility and accountability for their contribution to the whole.

In the zero-sum world of healthcare budgeting, a change in one department must be balanced with an equal and opposite change elsewhere. Department managers must understand how their unit statistics interact with strategic and financial assumptions to generate the target budget. They must communicate, in quantitative and measurable terms, any issues that would invalidate the first-pass budget.

The first round of budget review is relatively short in duration and results in the identification of any adjustments necessary to account for special situations. Items not identified as needing adjustment at this stage will remain unchanged unless truly extenuating circumstances occur. Thus, department managers must not hesitate to raise real issues or concerns at this point.

Step 6: Make adjustments and finalize the budget

Working with department managers, the finance team is able to adjust the budget to reflect the financial effect of issues and alternatives. The budget may then be finalized. This step occurs approximately one month before the final budget is submitted for board approval. It should not take longer than a month because it focuses solely on those departments with issues that represent significant changes from the first-pass budget. Managers of departments in which statistics, such as costs per unit or full-time equivalents (FTEs), are stable or improving know that they are done with the budgeting process and will not need to revise data.

Step 7: Use the budget as a management tool

In a best practice approach to financial management, the budget is an active tool for day-to-day management. It provides very precise guidance to all levels of the organization and is used on a regular basis. At the departmental level, monthly variance analysis assumes expanded meaning. Cost overruns or revenue shortfalls are evaluated in the context of overall organizational goals.

The connection between the budget and the organization's strategic financial plan must remain active throughout the year. Therefore, on a periodic basis (perhaps quarterly), executives and financial managers need to assess year-to-date performance not only against budget but also against the long-range financial plan. They should ask questions such as the following:

- How does the 3 percent negative variance from budget after the first quarter affect the organization's ongoing ability to continue to generate the capital capacity needed to support its strategic initiatives?
- What operating changes must be made during this fiscal year to ensure that the organization meets its long-term financial and strategic objectives?

Thus, the strategic budget becomes a living, organic document, providing guidance and analytical direction for the organization's daily operations. In

---

SIDEBAR 5-3. Sample Time Frame for an Integrated Budgeting Process

An integrated budgeting process shortens the actual budget development phase by half, running from March 1 through mid-May.

For a fiscal year running from July through June, completion dates might look like the following:

- December 1: Complete strategic plan.
- February 1: Complete financial plan.
- February 15: Define financial expectations for next annual budget.
- March 1: Develop and distribute budgets for/to each department.
- April 1: Department managers review budgets.
- May 15: Annual budget finalized.

Source: Kaufman, Hall & Associates, Inc. Used with permission.

---

contrast, for many organizations using the more common approach to budgeting described at the outset of this chapter, at this point the budget becomes an artifact relegated to the back shelf. Although the finance department generates monthly responsibility reports, no specific or discernible management decisions appear to result from the analysis.

Step 8: Restart the cycle

After the close of one fiscal year, the cycle recommences. At Step 1, executives review and update the organization's strategic plan. Steps 2 through 6 follow.

The schedule of the best practice approach to financial management must be rigorously followed to ensure the organization's ability to make consistent and timely decisions. Sidebar 5-3 illustrates a sample time frame in which the entire budgeting process is performed within several months.

Best Practice Strategic Budgeting Tools

Because today's market requires timely decision making, efficient, integrated, high-quality, and sophisticated budgeting software is critical. The

> ### SIDEBAR 5-4. Key Characteristics of Strategic Budgeting Software
>
> - *Flexibility*: The software must address the variety of operations within today's healthcare organization.
> - *The ability to evolve*: The software must be able to grow with the needs of the organization and deliver over the long term.
> - *Calculating power*: Healthcare budgeting is built on numerous and varied calculations, ranging from unit volumes to fixed and variable expenses to complex compensation structures. The software must easily accommodate each type of calculation.
> - *Security*: Management must be able to control distribution and access to the confidential information and detailed calculations supported by the software.
> - *Analytical capability*: The software must be able to integrate the strategic and financial planning processes with the budgeting process.
> - *Flexible reporting*: State-of-the-art software must support totally flexible reporting. From basic responsibility reporting to reporting of cost variance explanations, the software must allow the user to "slice and dice" the data to create management reports that focus on the issues at hand.
> - *Ease of use*: To achieve the broad-based use critical for an integrated best practice approach, the software must be easy to use. It must be comfortable and sturdy, thereby ensuring that new users are not afraid of "breaking it."
> - *Ease of maintenance*: After the software is installed, maintenance should be minimal and easily accomplished on an ongoing basis.
>
> Source: Kaufman, Hall & Associates, Inc. Used with permission.

tools that worked to support the budgeting process in healthcare organizations ten years ago are simply inadequate to meet the needs of today's complex organizations. Contemporary software must offer a wide range of benefits to support a best practice budgeting process, including flexibility, the ability to evolve, calculating power, security, analytical capability, flexible reporting, ease of use, and ease of maintenance (see Sidebar 5-4).

Through each of these characteristics, budgeting software ensures the integrity of the budgeting approach and thus the organization's confidence in the budgeting process. As described, decentralized decision making and accountability are key to the success of best practice strategic budgeting.

Tools that enable managers to fully understand the implications of their decisions and measure their outcomes help achieve the level of buy-in needed for a successful budgeting process.

The Benefits of Strategic Budgeting

A best practice strategic budgeting process incorporates budgeting as an integral part of the financial management cycle. All managers are educated about the organization's overall strategic imperatives—both market and financial—and are responsible for achieving those imperatives at the departmental level. This improved process emphasizes the importance of each operational component to the success of the whole organization. It is inclusive and flexible, yet quantitatively driven within specific rules and timing. It limits budget iterations and negotiations, yet is active and participatory.

In short, use of a best practice budgeting process helps executives ensure a direct link between their strategic and financial plans and day-to-day operations. This link is critical to the future success of healthcare organizations.

Case Example: Strategic Budgeting in Practice

This example describes one organization's recent implementation of a best practice budgeting process. This process provided a framework to operationalize the organization's strategy on a day-to-day basis. Although the name of the organization is fictitious, the information provided is real.

The organization at a glance

Part of a faith-based national health system, ABC Healthcare is a regional system serving the approximately 1.2 million residents of a major metropolitan area and its surrounding county. Generating more than $600 million in annual revenue, ABC Healthcare includes four acute care hospitals, physician clinics, a skilled nursing facility, a college of nursing, and numerous other entities.

Past budgeting approach

Before implementing the best practice approach to budgeting, ABC Healthcare's budgeting process was segmented and extremely complicated. "Because ABC Healthcare included multiple hospitals and other types of organizations, the finance team had to work with numerous different general ledger systems, accounting structures, and budgeting processes," notes the director of budget and decision support, who managed the implementation of the strategic budgeting process.

Under the past budgeting approach, the finance staff provided the 210 department directors with a series of volume worksheets, revenue worksheets, FTE worksheets, and operating expense worksheets. Each step of the budgeting process involved a two- to three-week time frame. The process was completely paper-based and required department managers to make manual mathematical calculations. After the managers submitted their worksheets, the finance staff had to key-in relevant data. "This was time consuming, and perhaps more importantly, because of the segmented nature of the data, the finance staff had to spend much more time entering data and reviewing the data for keying errors rather than analyzing the results. 'Big picture' analysis of the completed budget suffered," says the budget director.

Implementing a best practice approach

ABC Healthcare implemented strategic budgeting in fiscal year 2005. A new organizationwide decision support system and best practice approach was implemented. Spreadsheet-based budgeting software connected to a database enabled the organization to move to a completely electronic budgeting system. Department managers received intensive training in use of the new budgeting tool, which was loaded onto their personal computers. Group sessions provided hands-on education about software functions and the new budget templates. One-on-one sessions with the finance staff followed.

"Spreadsheet-astute department managers started serving as champions with their peers, making it easier to ensure rapid organizationwide integration of the new tool," says the budget director.

From strategic plan to financial targets

The best practice strategic budgeting approach engaged ABC Healthcare's executives and operations staff in making the budget process an integral part of the financial management cycle. Working with a July 1 through June 30 fiscal calendar, executives completed strategic plans by December 1 of each year. By this date, executives also developed or fine-tuned a multiyear financial plan that identified financial performance targets for the next annual budget within the context of ABC Healthcare's long-term strategic financial requirements. The leadership team created overall volume projections for the coming fiscal year, focusing on global statistical data such as total patient days, discharges, lengths of stay, outpatient visits, and physician clinic visits. The financial services department developed relationships as a result of tying these overall data to each department's primary statistic, as described earlier in this chapter.

Review of financial targets

During a budget environmental assessment meeting, department managers reviewed the strategic plan assumptions to validate the operational practicality of the plan goals. "In my estimation, this was the high point of the budget process, because it gave managers a look at the overall whole and the opportunity for input into the assumptions and the data that would drive the initial volume projections," notes the budget director. The group discussed, on a department-by-department basis, what might help achieve the goals of the strategic plan or prevent the plan's success. "The synergy created in that room was priceless—it put everyone on the same page and enabled all managers to clearly define the interdepartment impacts of defined strategic initiatives."

For example, when the director of oncology mentioned that a new oncology practice would be moving into an ABC Healthcare clinic and that he expected patient volume to increase by x percent, the pharmacy director stated that she would need to increase her budget for chemotherapy agents. The laboratory manager also noted volume changes that would need to be made to his budget. "The old budgeting process, characterized by managers 'doing their own thing,' was replaced by an interactive, integrated process," comments the budget director.

After this meeting, the budget director met with senior executives to summarize information provided by the department managers. Findings included the following:

- Length of stay, which had been decreasing steadily in one hospital due largely to a new surgical procedure performed in its major orthopedics unit, was starting to level off. The initial length-of-stay projections, which drove patient-day projections, needed to be adjusted upward for this facility. In addition, the finance staff recognized that length-of-stay projections could more accurately be made by service line rather than by the facility as a whole.
- Additional capacity was available at one facility because certain types of cases were shifting from inpatient to outpatient treatment. Admissions projections could be bumped up because of the facility's ability to handle more admissions.

Executives then modified volume projections, as needed, and closed the feedback loop by providing department managers with final financial targets.

Review of the first-pass budget

Next, in the first week of February, every department manager received an electronically distributed budget. Standardized budget templates displayed unique entity structure and data. Color coding identified areas requiring input by the department manager. Global assumptions were built into the templates.

For example, the manager of the surgery department received a report that translated global assumptions about targeted increases in overall admissions to the department's two key statistics—inpatient surgical cases and outpatient surgical cases. Hence, the department manager's volume budget was already completed, and he had only to verify the data.

"Managers loved the electronic files because most of the math was done for them. They just needed to review the results after inputting a few additional values," says the budget director. When projecting salary dollars, for example, department managers provided FTE information only, focusing solely on the number of people required to meet the projected volume level. The finance staff used budgeting software formulas to convert the FTEs to the appropriate hours and dollars data. The finance staff projected supply costs based on a variable cost basis plus an inflation factor. As volume changed, supply costs would go up or down appropriately. Department managers were able to adjust the inflationary increase if they knew price increases were going to exceed the inflation factor. For example, knowing that the nationwide industry average for pharmaceutical price increases was 5 percent to 13 percent, the finance staff used 8 percent as the inflationary increase. The pharmacy director could adjust this, as needed, and enter a comment about the basis for the adjustment in an appropriate narrative section for this item.

The new process also provided an opportunity for managers to raise any key concerns at this early budget development stage. "Knowing that the goal was to get the budget done in one-and-a-half passes, everyone worked hard to get the numbers right during the first pass. The big-ticket items were on the table, discussed, and agreed upon early on," notes the budget director. This eliminated the need for the repeated back-and-forth passes that are so prevalent with a typical budgeting approach.

Budget finalization

The financial services department finalized the budgets in March, focusing only on those issues that popped up on the radar screen. One such issue was "FTE creep." This occurred because department managers were budgeting for FTEs based on head count rather than actual staffing needs. For example, if five people were currently working in a specific department, the manager would override the 4.2 FTE count based on year-to-date actual data and insert 5 FTEs. To reconcile this problem, the finance staff talked with department managers about the realism of being at 100 percent staffing all year.

"The vast majority of the managers realized that 100 percent staffing would not be achieved throughout the year and backed off the higher FTE numbers," says the budget director. These managers, and those with flat or declining cost-per-unit of service or FTEs, were finished with the budgeting process—and it was only March. Budgets were compared to financial plan targets, and differences were reconciled.

A close look at a payroll summary for the surgery department illustrates the level of customized detail available within the budget database (Figure 5-1). The approach used in this monthly responsibility report involves tracking trends rather than the usual comparison of year-to-date and actual data. The display of biweekly payroll information allows the manager to more effectively review such issues as transfers between departments and time-code keying. "Because salary costs account for such a high percentage of the total organizational costs, close analysis of clean payroll data is critical," asserts the budget director.

Ongoing management

Managers use ABC Healthcare's budget in the daily management of operations. Each month, department managers receive electronically distributed responsibility reports the day after the month-end close. Figure 5-2 provides one page of the monthly departmental budget variance report for the surgery department. Year-to-date results are used to update current year and long-term financial plan projections.

Lessons learned

Within a one-year time frame, ABC Healthcare successfully implemented the numerous steps of a best practice budgeting process. The organization effectively rolled the financial plan down through the organization, learning the following lessons in the process:

- *Budgeting must be integrated into the whole of the financial management cycle.* Without this interconnectedness, ABC Healthcare would not have been able to operationalize its strategic and financial objectives.
- *Department managers must be informed of strategic financial targets and buy into such targets.* Best practice budgeting at ABC Healthcare transferred responsibility for the strategic plan's success down to the department manager level. Managers no longer received simple budget sheets with a request to input their wish lists. Instead, through the budget environmental assessment, managers were responsible for reviewing a budget

FIGURE 5-1. Surgery Department Payroll Summary

Department Payroll Summary—By Job Code
Pay Period Ending Date

Job Code Description	GL Code	FY05 PP-4 Budget Dollars	8/10/04 PP-3 Dollars	8/24/04 PP-4 Dollars	FY05 YTD—Actual Dollars	FY05 YTD—Budget Dollars
5203 Director surgical service	7010	0	0	0	6,899	0
5207 Materials manager surg	7010	2,230	2,236	2,236	8,944	8,760
5003 Nurse manager	7010	673	608	675	2,633	2,645
Total GL Code—7010		**2,903**	**2,844**	**2,911**	**18,476**	**11,405**
6506 Coord Surgery Info Syst	7020	1,656	1,661	1,661	6,643	6,507
Total GL Code—7020		**1,656**	**1,661**	**1,661**	**6,643**	**6,507**
5000 RN (Entry)	7030	0	1,627	1,513	6,288	0
5997 RN (Entry-surg)	7030	1,504	0	0	0	5,909
5001 RN (Experienced)	7030	0	1,756	1,756	7,024	0
5998 RN (Experienced-surg)	7030	47,327	35,298	34,191	139,916	185,926
5002 RN (Expert)	7030	0	1,947	2,294	8,403	0
4999 RN (Expert-surg)	7030	0	2,149	1,980	8,200	0
5023 RN Operating room Ed	7030	1,850	1,864	1,864	7,457	7,268
95001 RN Pool (Hosp)	7030	0	0	0	192	0
94998 RN Pool (Hosp-surg)	7030	18	24	168	576	72
5213 Surg Service Spec Coor	7030	12,218	14,541	14,630	57,760	47,999
Total GL Code—7030		**62,917**	**59,206**	**58,396**	**235,816**	**247,174**

Continued

FIGURE 5-1. Surgery Department Payroll Summary (continued)

Department Payroll Summary—By Job Code
Pay Period Ending Date

Job Code Description	GL Code	FY05 PP-4 Budget Dollars	8/10/04 PP-3 Dollars	8/24/04 PP-4 Dollars	FY05 YTD—Actual Dollars	FY05 YTD—Budget Dollars
00156M Anesthesia mntr tech	7050	0	0	945	945	0
95206 Surg tech/Asst pool	7050	13	0	149	537	52
5216 Surgical tech extern	7050	0	1,296	937	4,817	0
5206 Surgical tech/Surgical assistant	7050	47,511	42,225	39,922	163,403	186,652
Total GL Code—7050		**47,542**	**43,521**	**41,953**	**169,702**	**186,704**
5313 Operating room assistant	7070	7,848	8,260	7,199	30,799	30,830
Total GL Code—7070		**7,848**	**8,260**	**7,199**	**30,799**	**30,830**
5205 Coord materials	7080	2,037	2,044	2,164	8,281	8,003
5307 Surgery scheduler	7080	3,004	2,958	3,036	11,718	11,803
Total GL Code—7080		**5,041**	**5,002**	**5,200**	**19,999**	**19,806**
Grand Total		**127,889**	**120,494**	**117,320**	**481,435**	**502,426**

Source: Kaufman, Hall & Associates, Inc. Used with permission.

FIGURE 5-2. Surgery Department Monthly Budget Variance Report

Departmental Payroll Summary—Job Code

Monthly Departmental Budget Variance Report

Account No./Account Description	Aug-04 Actual ($)	Actual Per Unit ($)	Aug-04 Budget ($)	Budget Per Unit ($)	Budget Variance ($)	Aug-03 Actual ($)	2004-2005 Annual Budget ($)
Statistics							
10 IP Surgical cases	534		576		(42)	613	3,480
20 OP Surgical cases	670		585		85	541	3,194
Total Statistic	**1,204**		**1,161**		**43**	**1,154**	**6,674**
3200 IP ancillary services	4,966,070		4,511,549		454,521	4,113,090	27,276,595
Total Inpatient Revenue	**4,966,070**	**9,299.76**	**4,511,549**	**7,832.55**	**454,521**	**4,113,090**	**27,276,595**
4200 OP ancillary services	1,698,865		1,679,589		19,277	1,381,008	9,174,368
Total Outpatient Revenue	**1,698,865**	**2,535.62**	**1,679,589**	**2,871.09**	**19,277**	**1,381,008**	**9,174,368**
Total Patient Revenue	**6,664,935**	**5,535.66**	**6,191,138**	**5,332.59**	**473,798**	**5,494,098**	**36,450,963**
Expenses							
7010 S&W-Management and exec lead	19,724	16.38	12,857	11.07	(6,867)	22,683	77,510
7020 S&W-General/Medical professional	18,017	14.96	(5,541)	(4.77)	(23,557)	198,799	(31,808)
7030 S&W-Registered nurse	261,937	217.56	278,632	239.99	16,695	241,652	1,635,356
7040 S&W-Clinical assistants and aides						30,656	—
7050 S&W-General/Clinical tech specialist	176,029	146.20	210,466	181.28	34,437		1,248,832
7070 S&W-Service workers	33,885	28.14	34,754	29.93	869		208,940
7080 S&W-Office and clerical	22,228	18.46	22,326	19.23	98	30,411	134,079
Total Salaries	**531,820**	**441.71**	**553,494**	**459.71**	**21,675**	**524,201**	**3,272,909**
7326 Resident and intern fees	36,671	30.46	31,372	27.02	(5,299)	—	188,232
Total Professional Fees-Medical	**36,671**	**30.46**	**31,372**	**27.02**	**(5,399)**	—	**188,232**

Source: Kaufman, Hall & Associates, Inc. Used with permission.

that met defined targets of organizational performance for new and ongoing strategic initiatives and raising issues about why the given budget might not work. Managers identified exceptions or needed changes to an original budget and defined alternatives that might exist to counteract those changes to keep the budget balanced.

• *Budget reports must be user friendly.* Departmental budgets and responsibility reports need to be designed for ease of understanding and use. ABC Healthcare's responsibility reports evolved from basic reports to very robust analytic tools that department managers could use on an ongoing basis. Rework was not necessary to create new reports because a properly designed tool could meet all of the varied reporting needs.

ABC Healthcare's budget director concluded that although all department managers may not have agreed with the motto, "Budgeting is fun," best practice budgeting was not complex, cumbersome, or time consuming for department managers. Managers admitted that the process was "not bad"—a major victory for any organization!

A special note of thanks to the ABC Healthcare's budget director who described how the organization implemented the best practice budgeting approach in a way that would be enlightening for other healthcare organizations.

CONCEPT SIX

Achieving the Right Capital Structure

Caps. Collars. Corridors. Synthetic leases. Forward-starting fixed payer swaps. REITs. Sale-leasebacks. Senior-subordinated debt.

What are these things? Where did good old "plain vanilla" fixed-rate bonds go? Many of today's financial offerings bear little resemblance to those of five years ago. New product offerings (and variations thereof) for healthcare organizations are emerging from Wall Street firms each and every month.

The management of debt portfolios by not-for-profit healthcare organizations has experienced a similar transformation. Gone are the days of borrowing money at a fixed interest rate for 30 years and retaining that debt to maturity. Capital structure management now demands that financial leaders pay attention to interest costs on a regular basis and manipulate the capital structure when opportunities emerge to lower overall capital costs and increase flexibility.

Overview of Capital Structure and the Benefits of Its Effective Management

Capital structure is the combination of debt and equity that funds an organization's strategic plan. All healthcare organizations, whether for-profit or not-for-profit, must raise capital to buy the assets required to meet their strategic objectives. No healthcare organization can fund its long-term growth strategy solely from reserves or even from a combination of reserves and operating cash flow. All hospitals and health systems must access the capital markets on a regular basis.

The effective management of capital structure requires focus on the type of debt incurred by the organization, the cost and terms of debt capital, its flexibility and risk, and its overall ability to support the organization's competitive position and financial performance.

A strategic and proactive approach to capital structure management, using the principles and techniques of corporate finance prevalent in the for-profit world, can differentiate not-for-profit organizations from their competitors. Organized properly in an organization of any size, a capital structure can be easily adjusted to take advantage of fluctuating interest rates and the changing shape of interest rate yield curves. Capital structures by themselves can lower the overall cost of capital and can maximize the return of assets versus the cost of liabilities. Perhaps, most importantly, over a ten-year to 20-year planning horizon, the quality of a hospital's capital structure can cost or save the organization millions of dollars. During at least the past several years, the creatively managed capital structure has clearly become a significant competitive advantage for many hospitals (see Sidebar 6-1).

To achieve the key benefits of effective capital structure management, including increased capital access, added flexibility, and lower overall cost of capital, capital structure leadership must be driven by a knowledgeable senior financial management team. In many organizations, that team is best chaired by the organization's CFO, who offers a coherent approach to capital structure and possesses technical financial skills. The CFO also ensures that the financial management team, other senior executives, and the board are knowledgeable about the capital structure approach and techniques and obtain high-quality investment banking, legal, and consulting assistance, as required.

Debt/Equity Financing and Traditional/ Nontraditional Financing

Capital comes in many forms, but when obtained from external sources, it is generally classified as either debt capital or equity capital. Most healthcare leaders struggle with the basic question, "Is there an optimal mix of debt and

> **SIDEBAR 6-1. Sample Competitive Advantages That Can Be Achieved Through Effective Capital Structure Management**
>
> Consider a hospital with total debt of $300 million. If the hospital's executives can lower the cost of capital by 1 percent, the hospital saves $3 million per year. Over a ten-year period, savings amount to a very significant $30 million. Most hospital executives would be hard-pressed to identify other improvement strategies that could yield that level of savings.
>
> Consider also the effect of such savings on competitive strategic financial position. Perhaps the hospital is located in a two-hospital town, and both hospitals have a similar level of debt. Hospital A, which has lowered its overall cost of capital to 3 percent, has a distinct competitive advantage over Hospital B, which is paying 4 percent or more. The lower the cost of capital, the more capital capacity will be available to fund strategic initiatives.
>
> Organizations with substantial cash reserves may be able to use debt to improve the organization's balance sheet. If annual interest costs on debt service payments are lower than annual earnings from cash reserves, a hospital can achieve a net *surplus return* on its balance sheet, defined as the difference between the annual return on investments and the annual cost of debt (Wafer 2005). Over time, incremental surplus returns plus incremental investment earnings on surplus returns can significantly increase debt capacity, thereby reducing the capital constraint and increasing capital access.
>
> Source: Kaufman, Hall & Associates, Inc. Used with permission.

equity financing, and, if so, what is it?" The mix depends on rating agency benchmarks and the organization's debt capacity and tolerance for risk. Risk tolerance varies by organization and should be discussed and agreed on in advance by an organization's board of directors and senior management team.

Three major categories of debt vehicles are available to healthcare organizations, depending on the credit ratings of or credit enhancement available to the organization: traditional public offerings, traditional private placements, and nontraditional vehicles (Wareham 2004).

Traditional publicly offered bonds and notes can be taxable or tax exempt and can have fixed or variable rates. A public offering means the debt is structured to be offered and sold by an underwriter to any party—individuals or institutions— that is interested in owning the bonds. Tax-exempt bonds are the most common form of debt for hospitals.

A *traditional private placement* is debt offered by a limited universe of lenders, typically banks, leasing or equipment companies, insurance companies, or other large institutions. It can be taxable or tax exempt and can carry either fixed or variable rates. These can be in the form of bonds, notes, loans, or leases.

Nontraditional vehicles are numerous, including receivables financing, off-balance-sheet options (for example, operating leases, sale-leasebacks, synthetic leases), real estate investment trusts (REITs), participating bonds, and subordinated securities. Again, these can be taxable or tax exempt, although the hurdles for tax exemption force most of the vehicles to be taxable. Healthcare providers access these nontraditional alternatives if they have no other options or are trying to preserve their debt capacity for traditional vehicles. These financing forms are sometimes used to finance stand-alone assets that are off-site or not required for an organization's core business. Figure 6-1 describes characteristics of four types of off-balance-sheet vehicles.

Evaluation criteria

When considering which traditional and nontraditional financing vehicles are appropriate for an organization's circumstances and credit position, healthcare executives should consider 12 factors (Wareham 2004):

1. *All-in borrowing rate*: This is the total cost of capital, including interest costs and ongoing fees involved with maintaining the financing.
2. *Costs of issuance*: Tax-exempt bonds typically have higher costs of issuance than do taxable bonds, but in either case, organizations should carefully evaluate these costs.
3. *When the money is needed*: The timing of when the hospital needs to spend the money may affect its choice of vehicle. Direct lending from banks and private placements can usually be secured the most quickly.
4. *Use of proceeds*: The tax status of the financing option depends on the tax status of the entity for which the financing is being sought.
5. *Credit position*: The credit available to an organization largely determines which vehicles it can access.

FIGURE 6-1. Characteristics of Off-Balance-Sheet Vehicles

	True Operating Lease	Synthetic Lease	Sale-Leaseback	Joint Venture (Master Lease)
Types of Assets	Equipment and real estate; new or existing	Equipment and real estate; only for new assets	Typically, real estate	Typically, real estate
Approach	Acts like traditional debt, but off balance sheet	Lessee takes depreciation as owner; effectively a medium-term revolver applied to longer-term assets	If previously owned property, must be a true operating lease; if previously a capitalized lease, ineligible for sale-leaseback treatment	Developer provides equity and financing based on host's minimum occupancy agreement and ground lease
Taxable vs. Tax-Exempt	Either	Either	Either; existing property may not be eligible for tax exemption	Typically taxable
Lease Payments	Includes amortization of underlying principal so payments are usually larger than those for a synthetic lease; can have escalators and annual fees; subject to Financial Accounting Standards Board (FASB)	Probably lowest if structured as interest only in lease payments; can have escalators and annual fees; subject to FASB	Includes amortization of underlying principal so payments are usually larger than those for a synthetic lease; can have escalators and annual fees; subject to FASB	Structured to meet developer minimum return; excess shared with host

Source: Kaufman, Hall & Associates, Inc. Used with permission.

6. *Document structure and underlying security requirements*: The weaker the credit, the more security is required. The underlying security required by some financing vehicles can limit an organization's ability to issue debt in the future.

7. *Covenants*: There are two basic categories of covenants—maintenance and incurrence. Maintenance covenants are routine requirements that the borrower must meet on an annual and sometimes quarterly basis—for example, the liquidity covenant of days cash on hand. Incurrence covenants are special requirements that must be met before undertaking a particular action—for example, sale or disposition of property. Organizations should always seek the least restrictive covenants possible.

8. *Principal amortization*: The amortization schedule for the financing vehicle is critical to cash flow and maintenance covenants.

9. *Interest rate risk*: The best course is to achieve a mix of fixed- and variable-rate debt that minimizes interest rate risk.

10. *Average useful life versus average maturity*: Tax-exempt financing rules require that projects eligible for tax exemption be specifically delineated in the documents that support the borrowing.

11. *Disclosure requirements*: Tax-exempt vehicles require organizations to provide prompt, accurate, complete, and continuing disclosure of certain financial and utilization information.

12. *Prepayment penalties and unwind provisions*. Different financing vehicles have different premiums or prepayment penalties associated with an early redemption date.

All capital decisions should support an organization's strategic plan, provide as much flexibility as possible given existing and pending laws or restrictions, involve the lowest overall cost for the risk of the asset and liability portfolios, and allow for future financing needs.

Policy and framework

Given differing credit positions and organizational tolerance for risk, many CFOs, treasurers, and other healthcare leaders are increasingly feeling the need for a broad debt management policy that outlines approved parameters for the financial transactions required to effectively manage capital structure. The capital markets, particularly the rating agencies, have recommended that organizations maintain a policy on the use of derivatives and other complex financing options, whose inherent risks may or may not be well understood by the management team and board. A comprehensive policy can provide a road map for capital structure management going forward. Sidebar 6-2 outlines elements that can be included in such a policy.

Fixed-Rate Debt and Variable-Rate Debt

Once the debt and equity mix and the traditional versus nontraditional financing decisions are made, the next question becomes, "Given a specified level of debt, what's the right mix of fixed-rate debt to variable-rate debt?" Selecting the appropriate relationship is one of the most important capital structure decisions an organization's financial executives will make. Again, every healthcare organization has a different appropriate mix based on such factors as bond ratings, availability of bond insurance, amount of free cash, investment policy, board attitude toward risk, and the changing shape of interest rate yield curves. Use of more than 50 percent variable-rate debt may even be acceptable when a hospital has a tradition of very strong liquidity and cash flow (Fitch Ratings 2005).

Achieving the right mix requires planning, timing, and proper execution. Yield curve developments since 2001 have provided alert financial executives with excellent opportunities. Hospitals and health systems that moved fixed-rate to variable-rate debt in 2001 and the subsequent years may have saved hundreds of thousands and even millions of dollars in interest payments.

In fact, review of fixed-rate and variable-rate interest cost yields indicates that since 1991, variable-rate interest costs have been lower, and often significantly lower, than fixed-rate costs. When the yield curve changes, attentive executives adjust the proportion of fixed to variable-rate debt accordingly. Interestingly enough, notwithstanding lower variable-rate costs since 2001, the number and dollar volume of fixed-rate debt issues have been more than double that of variable-rate issues. However, a constant, but limited group of issuers has been taking advantage of the lower-cost variable-rate market (Kaufman 2005).

SIDEBAR 6-2. Elements of a Comprehensive Debt Management Policy

Principles/Scope and Authority
- Overall debt management objectives
- Scope of the policy, such as debt, lease financing, swaps, and other derivative products
- Policy review and approval process and administration authority

Analytical Requirements
- Credit rating goals and targets
- Elements of the long-range strategic financial plan related to debt issuance and debt service requirements
- Specific requirements of debt strategy, including asset/liability management analysis, analysis of diversification of financing vehicles, and management of specified risks

Approved Financial Products
- Debt and derivative instruments
- Process for adding or deleting specific instruments

Debt Policy
- Use of long-term debt, short-term debt, variable-rate debt, lease financing, real estate financing, and guaranties
- Qualified credit banks
- Purpose of new money financing and refunding bonds
- Approved uses of credit enhancement
- Responsibility for maintaining capital market relationships and continuing disclosure

Derivatives Policy
- Overall philosophy and rationale for using derivative products
- Required risk analysis and risk limits
- Appropriate derivative counterparties
- Authority for derivatives management

Source: Sussman, J. 2005. "Managing Capital Structure Through a Comprehensive Debt Management Policy." *The KaufmanHall Report*, Summer. Used with permission of Kaufman, Hall & Associates, Inc.

Choosing the correct mix of different variable-rate products is also a high-priority task for the hospital treasury function. Diversification of the variable-rate debt portfolio can consistently lower the organization's overall cost of capital. A diversified program could include variable-rate demand bonds backed by a bank letter of credit; insured auction rate securities; uninsured auction rate securities; investment banker proprietary products such as "direct lending" or "direct funding;" and, in the cases of the strongest credits, unenhanced variable-rate demand bonds.

A high-quality, variable-rate debt program avoids excessive exposure to any one form of risk, including the following:

- *Basis*: Risk that results from interest rate variance.
- *Put*: Risk that bonds can be "put" back to the hospital by the lender.
- *Bank*: Risk that renewal of a bank letter or proof of credit will come at an inopportune time or be unobtainable for a variety of reasons.
- *Credit*: Risk that an organization's credit rating changes while it is using certain programs that are dependent on the organization being at a certain credit level.
- *Failed auction*: Risk that occurs when there are more sellers of an issuer's paper on an auction date than there are buyers, and the whole offering is not resold.

Careful examination and monitoring of the organization's variable-rate program should allow the organization to achieve the lowest cost of capital possible at levels of risk acceptable to senior management and the board.

Swaps and Other Derivatives

A *derivative* is any sort of contract that manages or adjusts the character of underlying securities, whether debt or equity. Derivatives enable hospitals to maintain a flexible capital structure and to make real-time adjustments to that structure as demanded by both the interest rate and competitive environments. Derivatives also permit appropriate matching of assets to liabilities as interest rate and stock market conditions change. As an organization's capital structure increases in complexity, the importance of the use of derivative strategies also increases.

Derivatives include interest rate swaps (described later); plain-vanilla caps, which can protect organizations from increases in floating rates above a strike price; chooser caps, which can protect organizations from interest rate spikes on a retroactive basis; collars, which can protect organizations from increases above a cap, but benefits are reduced if rates decline below a floor; corridors, which can protect organizations from increases within a range of interest rates between two strike prices; and knockout caps, which can protect organizations from increasing interests rates up to a threshold where the cap "knocks out."

Heavily used by hospitals, derivatives come in every imaginable style and flavor. This is both good and bad news: good in that it provides more options to solve specific interest-rate management issues; bad in that it becomes more difficult for healthcare financial executives and board members to determine which trades are appropriate for the organization and which trades are speculative or may subject the hospital to excessive risk. An active derivative program requires active management and a high level of knowledge and independent expertise on the part of hospital or system management. Large dollars are at stake. Notes one rating agency, "Used without a coherent strategy or by borrowers with finances that are already vulnerable, such financial products can result in adverse credit consequences" (Fitch Ratings 2005).

One type of derivative—an *interest rate swap*—is a contract between two parties to exchange interest rate modes on a specific amount and type of debt. In the healthcare world, the hospital borrower is one counterparty, and a commercial or investment bank is the other counterparty. Swaps are not new. They are common tools of treasury management in the private sector and are becoming increasingly common in the public/not-for-profit sector (Wareham and Majka 2003). Swaps offer a means of synthetically changing the fundamental interest rate characteristics of debt; but, importantly, swaps and derivatives are financial products, *not* debt. Like other contracts, they can be reversed at any time, but like bonds, the value of the contracted trade changes as interest rates go up and down.

There are three basic types of interest rate swaps: fixed payer swaps, fixed receiver swaps, and basis swaps (see Figure 6-2). A description of each follows.

Fixed payer swaps convert variable-rate debt to fixed-rate debt. A hospital with variable-rate debt contracts with a swap counterparty to provide fixed payments over the life of the swap in exchange for receiving variable payments based on a defined index. The economics depend on the *term* of

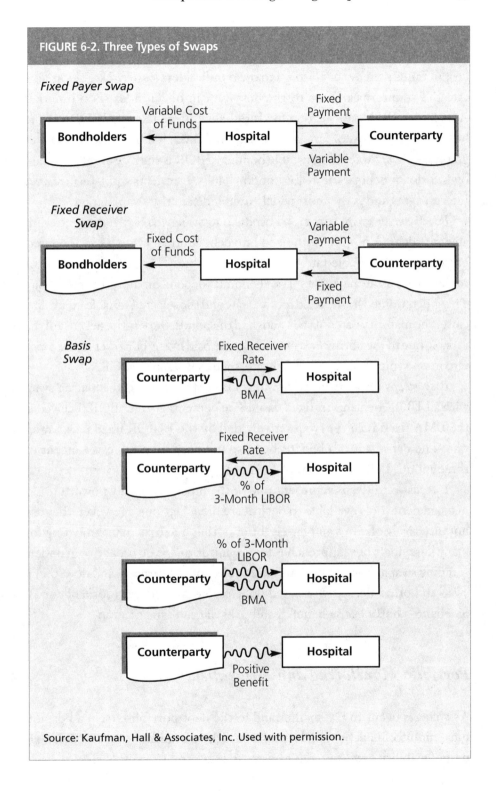

FIGURE 6-2. Three Types of Swaps

Source: Kaufman, Hall & Associates, Inc. Used with permission.

the swap. This is determined by the fixed payer rate and by the difference between the variable payment from the counterparty and the actual variable cost of funds paid by the hospital to the bondholders *(basis risk)*. The variable rate the counterparty pays to the hospital can be an index (Bond Market Association [BMA] or the London Interbank Offered Rate [LIBOR]) or the hospital's actual cost of funds. Set weekly, the BMA index is a proxy for high-grade *tax-exempt* weekly adjustable bonds. LIBOR is the rate of interest paid on U.S. dollar deposits at major London banks. It reflects short-term *taxable* interest rates and is the most widely used index in the swap market.

Fixed receiver swaps convert a hospital borrower's fixed-rate debt into variable-rate debt. A hospital with fixed-rate debt contracts with a swap counterparty to provide variable-rate payments over the life of the swap in exchange for receiving fixed-rate payments. The economics depend on the term of the swap. This is determined by the fixed receiver rate and the selected variable index. The closer the maturity dates of the swaps and the bonds, the less the net cost of the variable rate to the borrower. The variable rate paid by the borrower to the counterparty is typically a market index rate, such as BMA or LIBOR.

Basis swaps result from combining a tax-exempt, fixed-to-floating swap with a LIBOR floating-to-fixed swap. The percentage of LIBOR received is the BMA fixed receiver swap rate divided by the LIBOR fixed payer swap rate. The net result is a benefit because the hospital receives a percent of three-month LIBOR and pays BMA.

Interest rate swaps represent one of the most financially powerful risk-management tools available to healthcare organizations. However, they are not intuitively obvious and have subtleties that make them intimidating for many. The single best approach is for organizations to be proactive in understanding swaps, framing how and where they might be used, and developing swap and other derivative-related policies and procedures (Jordahl 2004). Sidebar 6-3 outlines the benefits and risks of each type of swap.

Portfolio Monitoring and Adjustment

As changes occur in the market and in the debt portfolio itself, a hospital must monitor its debt vehicles and adjust them regularly to maintain maximum flexibility, lowest possible costs, and acceptable levels of risk.

SIDEBAR 6-3. Benefits and Risks of Swaps		
Swap Type	**Benefits**	**Risks**
Fixed Payer	• Locks in fixed rates quickly and for little cost. If rates go up, the swap has positive value to the hospital • Enables hospital to add fixed-rate debt without actually issuing true fixed-rate debt • Provides greater budget predictability • May provide a closer match between assets and liabilities • Could allow for investment of bond proceeds at the higher fixed rate	• May require additional covenants or potential posting of collateral. Healthcare organizations should keep in mind with all types of swaps that commercial banks as counterparties do not typically require collateral • Required mark-to-market accounting treatment may not be favorable • Basis risk could be sizable unless there is an exact swap of a hospital's cost of funds • Potential cost (or benefit) from early termination • Counterparty's credit risk may be problematic
Fixed Receiver	• Under current market conditions, can provide interest cost savings • Can better match interest income with interest expense (assets to liabilities) • Because there is no exposure to bank credit facilities, eliminates renewal or price inflation risk and the need to negotiate covenants with a bank • Eliminates the hospital's exposure to event risk • Depending on timing, this type of swap can allow for the investment of bond proceeds at the higher fixed rate • Can be managed, which enables the hospital to benefit from market changes	• All-in variable payments may exceed the underlying fixed rate due to variable-rate risk and tax risk • Because the Bond Market Association index is reset on a weekly basis, the variable-rate portion of the swap may move in a direction unfavorable to the hospital • The credit risk of the counterparty may be problematic • Additional covenants or potential posting of collateral may be required • Potential cost (or benefit) from early termination • Mark-to-market accounting may not be favorable
Basis	• Can provide an immediate annual cash flow benefit, based on the relative value of the floating rate indexes • Can act as a hedge against higher tax-exempt variable rates by using a taxable index; as interest rates increase, so does the positive benefit • As marginal tax rates increase, cash flow benefits can improve • Under current market conditions, would provide interest cost savings	• Potential cost (or benefit) from early termination • Accounting treatment • Potential covenants and collateral posting • Credit risk of the counterparty • Cash flow benefit of basis swaps can decrease or become negative if marginal tax rates decrease and/or the supply of tax-exempt floaters increases

Source: Kaufman, Hall & Associates, Inc. Used with permission.

For example, many hospitals neglect the fairly simple mathematical principle that over time, the lowest NPV of total debt service payments will be accomplished by a level debt structure with the longest possible final maturity. The amortization period for bonds that produces the lowest NPV of payments is 30 years for many hospitals, and some hospitals and systems are extending this out even further. The average life of a 30-year bond issue is generally between 18 years and 20 years. As capital structures are built, however, amortization schedules that are not monitored carefully tend to "shorten up," and total annual payments become uneven. When this occurs, the hospital is paying off debt more quickly than it should, accelerating cash outflows and increasing total NPV of payments on the debt. Organizations with a higher-than-needed NPV of debt service payments that also simultaneously experience operating problems can run into serious cash flow and balance sheet difficulties.

Capital market and competitive environment changes make it critical for healthcare organizations to continuously monitor capital structure and every other aspect of the capital management cycle. Charts, calendars, and more sophisticated analytical tools are essential, as is expert advice. High-quality capital structure management, in effect, is increasing the gap between those hospitals with access to low-cost capital and those without such access. Although operating margins have improved for many healthcare organizations in the past few years, no organization can afford to neglect the pursuit of proactive strategies to lower the cost of capital. Capital structure is a hot-button financial issue that must receive careful and expert management attention.

References

Fitch Ratings. 2005. *Investment and Debt Portfolio Trends of Hospitals and Health Care Systems—1995-2003*. New York: Fitch Ratings.

Jordahl, E. A. 2004. "Nine Things to Know About Interest Rate Swaps." *The KaufmanHall Report* Fall: 1-4.

Kaufman, K. 2005. "Trends in Healthcare Debt Access." *Executive Insights* 3 (6): 1–3.

Sussman, J. 2005. "Managing Capital Structure Through a Comprehensive Debt Management Policy." *The KaufmanHall Report*, Summer.

Wafer, S. 2005. Personal communication with the author on 12/05/05. Note: The concept of surplus return, as applied to healthcare organizations, was first articulated by Steve Wafer of nProfit, LLC.

Wareham, T. L. 2004. "A Capital Idea: Bonds and Nontraditional Financing Options." *Healthcare Financial Management* 58 (5): 54–62.

Wareham, T. L., and A. J. Majka. 2003. "Best Practice Financing." White Paper. Northfield, IL: Kaufman, Hall & Associates, Inc.

CONCLUDING COMMENTS

Corporate Finance—A New Management Paradigm for Healthcare Organizations

ALTHOUGH THE RATING agencies forecast some stability in the healthcare sector in the short term, they cite numerous factors that could lead to longer-term credit risk and restricted access to capital. Clearly, the industry is caught between free market capitalism, which is characterized in many markets by hypercompetition, and escalating clinical and payment regulations. One force pushes revenues down; the other pushes costs up. The results speak for themselves.

Healthcare organizations need to recognize that more has changed here than just Medicare reimbursement. Gone are the years of pursuing strategic missions centered on improving health in local communities without a financially sound business plan that generates a profitable bottom line. The healthcare industry has crossed over from a public, mission-driven operating model to an operating model that closely resembles that of corporate America. The model is dominated by both the good and the bad aspects of the free-market economy.

A managerial response that is equal to the magnitude of the industry's financial problems is now required. The most obvious solution is to look to management models used by the companies that survive, and thrive, in this free-market jungle every day. The predominant management style is informed and driven by the corporate finance techniques described throughout this book. This style has defined the success of the GEs and Microsofts of the world.

Managing through corporate finance requires a change in technique and attitude. The managerial issues involved are straightforward.

Cost

Pressure on price is a constant of the free market. The only acceptable response is constant cost management. This involves reducing costs to the lowest possible level consistent with quality standards and customer service excellence and maintaining this level without fail. Cost management must be an ongoing approach supported by hospital leadership. Episodic and crisis cost control, which offers only a Band-Aid approach to financial problems, has proven to be entirely ineffective.

Goals and Objectives

As described in Concept Three, corporate finance techniques should be used to establish appropriate strategic and financial goals for the organization. These ensure the organization's ability to pursue its mission. At GE, the rhythm of financial planning is owned by financially educated managers all the way to the top. This gives the company what former chairman Jack Welch described in a 1995 shareholders letter as "all the strengths of a big company while moving with the speed, hunger and urgency of a small company." Goals and objectives should be quantified and ratified by the board. Next, they should be distributed widely throughout the organization. Objectives are hard to meet if they remain a closely held secret.

Accountability

Senior management must be accountable for successful financial performance. Leaders must reward achievement. Executives and trustees must not be so committed to consensus management models that no one is actually responsible for reaching short-term and long-term financial targets.

Measurement

"What gets measured gets done" is an often-cited message, but it is actually more complicated. GE has made the Six Sigma program one of its central

---

SIDEBAR CC-1. What Is Six Sigma?

First, what Six Sigma is not: it is not a secret society, a slogan, or a cliché. Six Sigma is a highly disciplined process that helps companies focus on developing and delivering near-perfect products and services. Why "Sigma?" The word is a statistical term that measures how far a given process deviates from perfection. The central idea behind Six Sigma is that if you can measure how many defects you have in a process, you can systematically figure out how to eliminate them and get as close to zero defects as possible.

Six Concepts of Six Sigma

1. Critical to quality: Attributes most important to the customer
2. Defect: Failing to deliver what the customer wants
3. Process capability: What the process can deliver
4. Variation: What the customer sees and feels
5. Stable operations: Ensuring consistent, predictable processes to improve what the customer sees and feels
6. Design for Six Sigma: Designing to meet customer needs and process capability

Source: Adapted from General Electric, "Quality" [Online information; retrieved 1/6/2006]. http://www.ge.com/en/company/companyinfo/quality/whatis.htm.

---

administrative principles (see Sidebar CC-1). At GE, this quality program is applied not only to manufacturing but to general operations and management. It is a way of life for all employees. The GE mnemonic is DMAIC: define, measure, analyze, improve, and control.

Calendar Management

Calendar management may seem unrelated to this discussion and to corporate finance, but it is very relevant. As outlined in Concept Four, calendar management describes the schedule and process an organization uses to create a comprehensive financial plan and defines the rigor with which leaders move important financial information through the organization. Calendar management defines the relationship between strategic planning, financial planning, the operating budget, and capital allocation (see Figure 4-1 in

Concept Four). Financial rigor and discipline are impossible without planning schedules that are obsessively followed and widely understood within the organization.

Allocation of Resources

The free market demands the careful, scientific, and quantitative allocation of resources. This is especially true of capital. Many healthcare organizations are now suffering from a history of allocating capital in a manner that was mostly casual and political. The assumption was that core businesses could generate sufficient cash flow to support investment initiatives that did not have acceptable returns. The best practice approach to capital allocation required in today's environment includes sound financial planning, review of all projects on a level playing field, coordinated calendar and planning cycles, and the use of corporate finance–based analytical concepts. Such concepts include determining the net cash available for capital, incremental cash flow projections, discounted cash flow or NPV, and weighted average cost of capital (see Concept Four).

Strategy and Capital

There must be a powerful link between strategy and capital investment. Strategy must be well thought out and well articulated. It must focus on external market needs and how the healthcare organization can best meet those needs. Strategic planning must precede financial planning, and both elements must be analytical, quantitative, and data driven. Critical proven strategies must be directly and aggressively supported by consistent investment.

Balance Sheet Management

Free-market success demands solid balance sheets. A corporate finance–driven organization's first instinct in a difficult market is to protect the integrity of its balance sheet. For not-for-profit hospitals, this means an adequate cash position, an appropriate amount of debt, the right capital structure, and a dependable credit rating that allows reasonable access to capital.

SIDEBAR CC-2. Practical Applications of Corporate Finance for Senior Management and Board Members

Managerial Issue	Behavior
Cost	Constant cost management, not cost control
Goals and objectives	Board sets quantitative goals and objectives
Accountability	Direct and unambiguous executive accountability for results
Measurement	Operating results are constantly measured against articulated goals and objectives
Calendar management	Rigorous, bureaucratic, and almost obsessive attention to calendar management
Allocation of resources	Scarce resources (such as capital) are allocated carefully and scientifically
Strategy and capital	There is a powerful link between capital investment and strategy
Balance sheet management	When things get difficult, a corporate finance organization's first instinct is to protect its balance sheet

Source: Kaufman, Hall & Associates, Inc. Used with permission.

Traditional hospital administration techniques will not adequately handle the unsentimental free-market economic conditions in today's healthcare world. America's highest performing organizations use corporate finance—not just as a set of analytic tools but as a coherent management style and philosophy (see Sidebar CC-2). The corporate finance activities of credit and capital structure, financial planning, capital allocation, and strategic budgeting can create a road map for financial success even in the most competitive and rigorous of free-market conditions.

Selected Bibliography

Books/Monographs

Baker, J. J., and R. W. Baker. 2006. *Health Care Finance: Basic Tools for Nonfinancial Managers, 2nd ed.* Sudbury, MA: Jones and Bartlett Publishers.

Berger, S. 2002. *Fundamentals of Healthcare Financial Management: A Practical Guide to Fiscal Issues and Activities, 2nd ed.* San Francisco: Jossey-Bass.

———. 2005. *The Power of Clinical and Financial Metrics: Achieving Success in Your Hospital.* Chicago: Health Administration Press.

Chew, D. H. 2001. *The New Corporate Finance: Where Theory Meets Practice, 3rd ed.* Boston: Irwin McGraw-Hill.

Cleverley, W. O., and A. E. Cameron. 2002. *Essentials of Health Care Finance, 5th ed.* Sudbury, MA: Jones and Bartlett Publishers.

Coile, R. 2002. *Futurescan 2002: A Forecast of Healthcare Trends 2002-2006.* Chicago: Health Administration Press.

Eastaugh, S. R. 2004. *Health Care Finance and Economics.* Sudbury, MA: Jones and Bartlett Publishers.

Gapenski, L. C. 2003. *Understanding Healthcare Financial Management, 4th ed.* Chicago: Health Administration Press.

———. 2004. *Healthcare Finance: An Introduction to Accounting and Financial Management, 3rd ed.* Chicago: Health Administration Press.

Ginter, P. M., L. E. Swayne, and W. J. Duncan. 2005. *Strategic Management of Health Care Organizations, 5th ed.* Malden, MA: Blackwell Publishers.

The Governance Institute. 2003. *The New Competitive Landscape: Board and CEO Strategies for Dealing with Emerging Threats.* San Diego, CA: The Governance Institute.

———. 2005. *Raising the Bar: Increased Accountability, Transparency, and Board Performance.* San Diego, CA: The Governance Institute.

Griffith, J. R., and K. R. White. 2002. *The Well-Managed Healthcare Organization, 5th ed.* Chicago: Health Administration Press.

———. 2003. *Thinking Forward: Six Strategies for Highly Successful Organizations.* Chicago: Health Administration Press.

Kemper, J. E. 2004. *Launching a Healthcare Capital Project: What Every Healthcare Executive Should Know.* Chicago: Health Administration Press.

Meyers, S. C., and R. A. Brealy. 2003. *Principles of Corporate Finance, 7th ed.* Boston: McGraw-Hill/Irwin.

Moody's Investors Service. 2000. *An Updated Approach to Rating Not-for-Profit Healthcare Organizations.* New York: Moody's Investors Service.

Nowicki, M. 2004. *The Financial Management of Hospitals and Healthcare Organizations, 3rd ed.* Chicago: Health Administration Press.

Pointer, D. D., and D. M. Stillman. 2004. *Essentials of Health Care Organization Finance: A Primer for Board Members.* San Franciso: Jossey-Bass.

Samuels, D. I. 1998. *Healthcare Financial Management Budgeting Toolkit.* Westchester, IL: Healthcare Financial Management Association.

Savage, S. L. 2003. *Decision Making with Insight, 2nd ed.* Pacific Grove, CA: Brooks/Cole, Thomson.

Society for Healthcare and Market Development and American College of Healthcare Executives. 2006. *Futurescan: Healthcare Trends and Implications 2005-2010*. Chicago: Health Administration Press.

Tyler, J. L., and E. Biggs. 2001. *Practical Governance*. Chicago: Health Administration Press.

Zelman, W. N., M. J. McCue, A. R. Millikan, and N. D. Glick. 2003. *Financial Management of Health Care Organizations: An Introduction to Fundamental Tools, Concepts, and Applications, 2nd ed*. Malden, MA: Blackwell Publishers.

Zuckerman, A. M. 2005. *Healthcare Strategic Planning, 2nd ed*. Chicago: Health Administration Press.

Recent Rating Agency, Industry, and Kaufman Hall Reports, White Papers, and Articles

HFMA. *Financing the Future I*. 2004. *How Are Hospitals Financing the Future: The Future of Capital Spending*. Westchester, IL: Healthcare Financial Management Association.

———. *Financing the Future II*. 2005. *Essentials of Integrated Strategic Financial Planning and Capital Allocation*. Westchester, IL: Healthcare Financial Management Association.

———. 2005. *Seven Principles of Best Practice Financial Management*. Westchester, IL: Healthcare Financial Management Association.

———. 2005. *Strategies for Effective Capital Structure Management*. Westchester, IL: Healthcare Financial Management Association.

Fitch Ratings. 2003. *Guidelines for Effective Uses of Swaps in Asset-Liability Management*. New York: Fitch Ratings, Feb 6, [Pamphlet].

———. 2005. *Healthcare Rating Actions for the Nine Months Ended Sept. 30, 2005*. New York: Fitch Ratings.

———. 2005. *Rating Process for Nonprofit Healthcare Credits*. New York: Fitch Ratings.

———. 2005. *Investment and Debt Portfolio Trends of Hospitals and Health Care Systems—1995-2003*. New York: Fitch Ratings.

Grube, M. E. 2004. "Finance's Role in Strategic Planning." *Executive Insights* 2 (7) 1–3.

Grube, M. E., and T. L. Wareham. 2005. "What Is Your Game Plan? Advice from the Capital Markets." *Healthcare Financial Management* 59 (11): 63–75.

———. 2005. *Essentials of Strategy: A Capital Markets Perspective*. Northfield, IL: Kaufman, Hall & Associates, Inc.

Hall, M. L. 2002. *Using Simulation Analysis to Improve Financial Decision Making*. Northfield, IL: Kaufman, Hall & Associates, Inc.

Jordahl, E. A. 2004. "Nine Things to Know About Interest Rate Swaps." *The KaufmanHall Report* Fall: 1-4.

Kaufman, F. 2005. *A Primer on Hospital Accounting and Finance*. Northfield, IL: Kaufman, Hall & Associates, Inc.

Kaufman, K. 1997. "Managing the Strategic Capital Cycle." *Healthcare Financial Management* 51 (12): 52–55.

———. 2000. *Corporate Finance: A New Management Paradigm*. Northfield, IL: Kaufman, Hall & Associates, Inc.

———. 2003. "Nine Observations on Credit Strategy for Not-for-Profit Hospitals." *Executive Insights* 1 (8): 1–3.

———. 2004. "Effective Financial Leadership: Walking the Walk vs. Talking the Talk." *Executive Insights* 2 (2): 1–3.

———. 2004. "Capital Structure: An Imperative Issue for Healthcare CFOs in 2005." *Executive Insights* 2 (12): 1–3.

———. 2005. "Trends in Healthcare Debt Access." *Executive Insights* 3 (6): 1–3.

Moody's Investors Service. 2004. "The Capital Spending Ratio" (Special Comment). New York: Moody's Investors Service.

———. 2005. *Indicators of Successful Management for Not-for-Profit Hospitals.* New York: Moody's Investors Service.

———. 2005. "Not-for-Profit Hospital-Physician Integration: New Strategies or Back to the Future?" (Special Comment). New York: Moody's Investors Service.

Standard & Poor's. 2005. *Turnaround Consulting Engagements: Assessing the Impact on U.S. Not-for-Profit Health Care Ratings.* New York: Standard & Poor's.

———. 2005. *U.S. Not-for-Profit Health Care 2005 Outlook: The Calm Before the Storm.* New York: Standard & Poor's.

———. 2005. *U.S. Not-for-Profit Health Care Sector Explores Benefits of Sarbanes-Oxley.* New York: Standard & Poor's.

Sussman, J. H. 2001. *Capital Allocation the Right Way: Consistent, Concurrent, Connected, and Communicated.* Northfield, IL: Kaufman, Hall & Associates, Inc.

———. 2002. *Strategic Budgeting: A Healthcare Imperative.* Northfield, IL: Kaufman, Hall & Associates, Inc.

Sussman, J. H., and M. E. Grube. 2003. *True Integration of Strategic and Financial Planning.* Northfield, IL: Kaufman, Hall & Associates, Inc.

———. 2004. "Joint Resolution: Blending Finance and Strategy." *Healthcare Financial Management* 58 (11): 42–50.

Wareham, T. L. 2001. "Strategies for Navigating the Healthcare Credit Market." *Healthcare Financial Management* 55 (4): 55.

———. 2004. "A Capital Idea: Bonds and Nontraditional Financing Options." *Healthcare Financial Management* 58 (5): 54–62.

———. 2005. "Seven Strategies for Achieving the Best Possible Bond Pricing." *Executive Insights* 3 (4): 1–3.

Wareham, T. L., and A. J. Majka. 2003. *Best Practice Financing.* Northfield, IL: Kaufman, Hall & Associates, Inc.

About the Authors

KENNETH KAUFMAN is managing partner of Kaufman, Hall & Associates, Inc. Founded in 1985, Kaufman Hall is an independent financial and capital consulting firm that provides financial advisory services and financial software to healthcare organizations of all types and sizes.

Since 1976, Mr. Kaufman has consulted to healthcare organizations throughout the country in the areas of strategic financial planning; capital planning and allocation; joint venture development; financial advisory services; and mergers, acquisitions, and divestitures. His focus is on helping healthcare executives improve the quality of their decision making and helping them ensure that their organizations become and stay financially competitive.

Mr. Kaufman has presented more than 200 educational programs to audiences throughout the United States, including seminars sponsored by the Healthcare Financial Management Association (HFMA), American College of Healthcare Executives (ACHE), American Hospital Association, and The Governance Institute. His audiences routinely include the top CEOs, CFOs, and board of director members from hospitals and health systems nationwide.

Mr. Kaufman's publications include five books — *The Capital Management of Health Care Organizations* (Health Administration Press, 1990), *The Financially Competitive Healthcare Organization* (HFMA/Irwin, 1994), the first edition of *Finance in Brief: Six Key Concepts for Healthcare Leaders* (Health Administration Press, 2000), the second edition (Health Administration

153

Press, 2003), and this third edition, now titled *Best Practice Financial Management: Six Key Concepts for Healthcare Leaders.* He has also written two white papers on healthcare financial management and more than 30 articles, which have appeared in most major healthcare publications, including *Healthcare Financial Management, Trustee, Modern Healthcare, BoardRoom Press, Frontiers of Health Services Management, and Hospitals & Health Networks.*

Mr. Kaufman holds a master's degree in business administration from the University of Chicago Graduate School of Business with a concentration in hospital administration. He is also a member of the board of directors of the Northwestern Medical Faculty Foundation.

JASON H. SUSSMAN is a partner of Kaufman, Hall & Associates, Inc. Mr. Sussman's experience includes all aspects of financial planning and financial advisory services for hospitals, healthcare systems, and physician groups. His areas of expertise include strategic financial planning, capital allocation, mergers and acquisitions, and various financing transactions.

Prior to joining Kaufman Hall, Mr. Sussman directed the Chicago Capital Finance Group of a national accounting firm's healthcare consulting practice. His consulting there related to assessment of financial feasibility, mergers and acquisitions, business plan development, and capital plan development. Mr. Sussman was the Special Assistant to the President at Michael Reese Hospital and Medical Center in Chicago, responsible for the Certificate of Need and capital budgeting processes at the institution, prior to his consulting experience.

Mr. Sussman has authored articles for various industry periodicals, including *Healthcare Financial Management*, and was a contributing author to *The Financially Competitive Healthcare Organizations, Finance in Brief: Six Key Concepts for Healthcare Leaders*, and *Topics in Health Care Finance.* He has presented programs at seminars sponsored by ACHE, the national HFMA, regional HFMA chapters, and NACHRI.

Mr. Sussman holds a Master of Management from Northwestern University's J. L. Kellogg Graduate School of Management in finance and accounting with a specialization in healthcare management, and a Bachelor of Arts Degree from the Johns Hopkins University. He has a CPA certificate in Illinois and is a member of the First Illinois chapter of HFMA and an Affiliate of the ACHE.